CLINICAL CARE

of the

Diabetic Foot

David G. Armstrong, DPM, MD, PHD
Lawrence A. Lavery, DPM, MPH

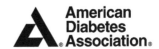

American
Diabetes
Association

Director, Book Publishing, Abe Ogden; *Managing Editor,* Greg Guthrie; *Acquisitions Editor,* Victor Van Beuren; *Project Manager,* Wendy M. Martin-Shuma; *Production Manager and Composition,* Melissa Sprott; *Cover Design,* Sport Creative; *Printer,* Data Reproductions Corp..

Printed in the United States of America
1 3 5 7 9 10 8 6 4 2

The suggestions and information contained in this publication are generally consistent with the *Standards of Medical Care in Diabetes* and other policies of the American Diabetes Association, but they do not represent the policy or position of the Association or any of its boards or committees. Reasonable steps have been taken to ensure the accuracy of the information presented. However, the American Diabetes Association cannot ensure the safety or efficacy of any product or service described in this publication. Individuals are advised to consult a physician or other appropriate health care professional before undertaking any diet or exercise program or taking any medication referred to in this publication. Professionals must use and apply their own professional judgment, experience, and training and should not rely solely on the information contained in this publication before prescribing any diet, exercise, or medication. The American Diabetes Association—its officers, directors, employees, volunteers, and members—assumes no responsibility or liability for personal or other injury, loss, or damage that may result from the suggestions or information in this publication.

Jane Chiang, MD, conducted the internal review of this book to ensure that it meets American Diabetes Association guidelines.

♾ The paper in this publication meets the requirements of the ANSI Standard Z39.48-1992 (permanence of paper).

American Diabetes Association titles may be purchased for business or promotional use or for special sales. To purchase more than 50 copies of this book at a discount, or for custom editions of this book with your logo, contact the American Diabetes Association at the address below or at booksales@diabetes.org.

American Diabetes Association
1701 North Beauregard Street
Alexandria, Virginia 22311

DOI: 10.2337/9781580405706

Library of Congress Cataloging-in-Publication Data

Clinical care of the diabetic foot / edited by David G. Armstrong, Lawrence A. Lavery. -- 3rd edition.
p. ; cm.
Includes bibliographical references and index.
ISBN 978-1-58040-570-6 (paperback)
I. Armstrong, David G., 1969-, editor. II. Lavery, Lawrence A., 1960-, editor. III. American Diabetes Association.
[DNLM: 1. Diabetic Foot. 2. Clinical Medicine--methods. WK 835]
RC951
617.5'85--dc23
                                    2015018693

"To my talented, beautiful better half, Tania,
and our lovely luminous ladies:
Alexandria, Natalie, and Nina (and Chloe)."
—D.G.A.

Contents

Foreword

"The era of coma has given way to the era of complications."
—Elliot P. Joslin

This quote, made in the first half of the last century by the late Professor Joslin, is as fitting today as it was 70 years ago. Our patients no longer die from acute conditions stemming from hyperglycemia. Rather, the chronic complications of the disease predominate. Chief among these complications is pathology related to the diabetic foot, which is the most common reason for hospital admission in people with diabetes. Only a generation ago, most clinicians considered it a fait accompli that once a person with diabetes developed lower-extremity complications, the end result would be an amputation, reamputation, and premature death. Over the past generation, care of the diabetic foot has matured from its previous state of nihilism into what is now a bona fide area of subspecialty and hope. It is now widely accepted that many lower-extremity complications of diabetes are preventable.

While many clinicians will appreciate that the diabetic foot is an area that deserves attention, most are so focused on and inundated with more proximal issues, that the myriad potential distal complications seem at once both daunting and beyond control. It is true that care of the diabetic foot spans the spectrum from surgery to endocrinology, from podiatry to infectious disease, from psychology to dermatology. It is to these clinicians to whom this book is dedicated.

This third edition refreshes data on screening, healing, and prevention.

Most notably, the comprehensive diabetic foot exam and rapid response systems are further articulated and outlined as "toe and flow," and other models of diabetic foot units become more common throughout the world.

We are honored and humbled to have worked with such a stellar group of clinician-scientists in the production of this work. This book assembles under one cover many of the people collectively responsible for transforming and advancing diabetic foot and wound care from its beginnings into its current state. This assembly will discuss nearly all aspects of care of the diabetic foot and wound and will do so in a practical, yet evidence-based manner.

To you, the reader, we extend an enthusiastic invitation to avail yourself of the collective wisdom of these contributors. It is our hope that this work stimulates you to investigate further what we believe is a fascinating and fruitful area of medicine. Enjoy.

David G. Armstrong, DPM, MD, PhD

Lawrence A. Lavery, DPM, MPH

1
Pathogenesis of Diabetic Foot Complications

Andrew J.M. Boulton, MD, DSc (Hon), FRCP
Manchester Royal Infirmary, Division of Medicine, Manchester, U.K.

Foot complications, which include foot ulceration, neuropathic osteoarthropathy (Charcot foot), and amputation, are common among patients with diabetes. It is estimated that >5% of these patients have a history of foot ulcers, and the cumulative lifetime incidence may be as high as 25%. Some 85% of all amputations are preceded by foot ulcers; therefore, reducing the incidence of foot ulcers should reduce the number of amputations as well.[1–3]

Risk Factors

Foot ulcers rarely result from a single pathology; two or more factors contribute. The neuropathic foot does not spontaneously ulcerate. Insensitivity combined with either extrinsic factors (such as walking barefoot and stepping on a sharp object or simply wearing ill-fitting shoes) or intrinsic factors (a patient with insensitivity and callus walks and develops an ulcer) ultimately results in ulceration. Neuropathy is the most important cause of ulceration.

Neuropathy

The association between both somatic and autonomic neuropathy and foot ulceration has long been recognized. However, only in the last decade have prospective follow-up studies confirmed the role of somatic neuropathy in causing foot ulcers. Patients with sensory loss appear to have up to a sevenfold increased risk of developing foot ulcers, compared with non-neuropathic diabetic individuals.[4] Poor balance and instability are increasingly being recognized as troublesome symptoms of peripheral neuropathy, presumably secondary to proprioceptive loss.

Peripheral autonomic (sympathetic) dysfunction results in dry skin and, in the absence of peripheral arterial disease, a warm foot with distended dorsal foot veins. However, because patients often think that all foot problems result from vascular disease, some may find it difficult to accept that their warm, but pain-free, feet are at significant risk of unperceived trauma and subsequent ulceration.

In practice, peripheral neuropathy can easily be determined by examining the foot for evidence of neuropathy—detailed quantitative sensory testing or electrophysiology is not needed. Simple tools such as a modified neuropathy disability score[4] and the monofilament may be used to help identify the at-risk neuropathic foot. (Additional details about the foot exam are provided in Chapter 2.)

Peripheral Arterial Disease

In approximately one-third of all cases, peripheral ischemia resulting from proximal arterial disease is a contributing factor in ulceration. The ischemic foot is red, dry, and often neuropathic, so it is susceptible to pressure from footwear.

Other Risk Factors

The presence of foot deformity, particularly claw toes and prominent metatarsal heads, is a proven risk factor for ulceration. Similarly, one cross-sectional study[5] showed that plantar callus accumulation was associated with an 11-fold increase in risk. During follow-up of these patients, plantar ulcers occurred only at sites of callus in neuropathic feet. Other risk factors include the presence of other microvascular complications, long duration of diabetes, increases in plantar foot pressures, and peripheral edema. More recent work has confirmed that diabetic patients with end-stage renal disease who are on dialysis are at very high risk of developing foot lesions[6]: both patients on dialysis and the medical staff on dialysis units need to be made aware of this. Most predictive of all was a past history of foot ulcers or amputation.

Prevention

Education

Preventing foot ulcers among individuals with risk factors is key to reducing the incidence of ulcers. Unfortunately, studies of preventive education have not confirmed its usefulness. Education along with regular podiatric care, however, may result in earlier presentation when ulcers develop.

A few studies have assessed psychosocial factors.[7] Patients' behavior is apparently not driven by being designated "at risk"—rather, it is driven by the patients' own perception of their risks. Thus, if patients believe that a foot ulcer could lead to amputation, they are more likely to follow educational advice on ways to reduce ulcer risk. Figure 1.1 outlines a pathway to foot ulceration, including areas where psychosocial factors are relevant. Additional research in this area is urgently required.

Foot Examinations

The most important aspect of diagnosing the foot at risk of ulceration is regularly asking patients to remove their shoes and socks and examining the foot in detail for evidence of neuropathy, vascular disease, deformities, plantar callus, edema, and other risk factors. A simple foot pressure mat (such as the PressureStat system; Foot Logic, New York) can help identify high pressures under the diabetic foot. Furthermore, these pressure maps of the foot, which show higher pressure areas as darker, may be used to educate patients about their risk for subsequent ulceration.

The Pathway to Ulceration

The combination of two or more of the risk factors discussed above ultimately results in diabetic foot ulceration. Various work[2,3,9] has suggested that the most common triad leading to breakdown of the diabetic foot includes peripheral neuropathy (insensitivity), deformity (clawing of the toes, prominence of metatarsal heads), and trauma (from footwear and/or repetitive stress). Other simple examples of a two-component pathway to ulceration are neuropathy and mechanical trauma (such as stepping on a nail) or neuropathy and thermal trauma (inappropriate use of chemical "corn cures" or when a patient with insensate feet uses a heating pack). Recent evidence suggests that

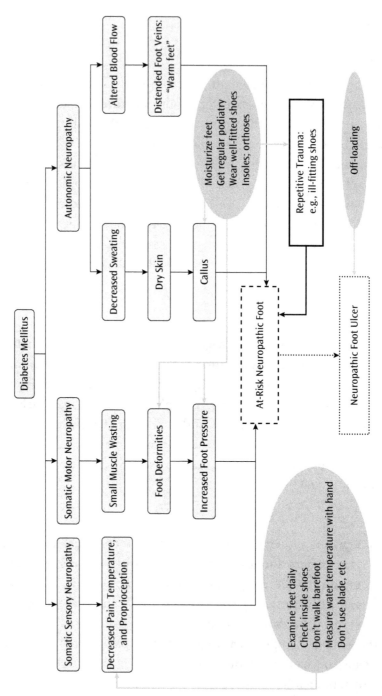

Figure 1.1—Causal pathways to foot ulceration, emphasizing the key role of the patient in ulcer prevention (spheres). From Boulton,[8] reprinted with permission.

the foot heats up just before ulceration, suggesting that skin temperature monitoring might provide an early warning of a pre-ulcerative lesion.[10]

The Patient with Sensory Loss

To reduce neuropathic foot problems, keep in mind that patients with insensitivity have lost the warning signal—pain—that ordinarily brings the patient to the doctor. Pain often leads to medical consultations, and our training and health care focus on the cause and relief of symptoms. Thus, the care of the patient with no pain sensation is a challenge for which we have little training. However, we can learn from those who treat leprosy, another disease in which patients' loss of pain diminishes their motivation to heal and prevent injury.

Charcot Neuroarthropathy

Charcot neuroarthropathy occurs in patients with peripheral loss of sensation and autonomic dysfunction (increased blood flow to the foot and dry skin), usually with unperceived trauma. The patient at risk of Charcot neuroarthropathy typically has a warm foot with bounding pulses but complete loss of sensation. Any patient presenting with unilateral warm, swollen foot, with or without symptoms of pain or discomfort, and good circulation should be considered to have Charcot neuroarthropathy until proven otherwise. (Chapter 9 discusses the presentation and management of Charcot neuroarthropathy.)

References

1. Singh N, Armstrong DG, Lipsky BA. Preventing foot ulcers in persons with diabetes. *JAMA* 2005;293:217–228

2. Boulton AJM. The diabetic foot: an update. *Foot Ankle Surg* 2008; 14:120–124

3. Boulton AJM. The pathway to foot ulceration in diabetes. *Med Clin N Am* 2013;97:775–790

4. Abbott CA, Carrington AL, Ashe H, et al. The North-West Diabetes Foot Care Study: incidence of, and risk factors for, new diabetic foot ulceration in a community-based patient cohort. *Diabet Med* 2002; 19:377–384

5. Murray HJ, Young MJ, Hollis S, Boulton AJ. The association between callus formation, high pressures and neuropathy in diabetic foot ulceration. *Diabet Med* 1996;13:979–982

6. Lavery LA, Lavery DC, Hunt NA, et al. Amputations and foot-related hospitalisations disproportionately affect dialysis patients. *Int Wound J* doi: 10.1111/iwj.12146. Epub 19 Sept 2013

7. Vileikyte L. Psychosocial and behavioral aspects of diabetic foot lesions. *Curr Diab Rep* 2008;8:119–125

8. Boulton AJM. The diabetic foot—from art to science: 18th Camillo Golgi Lecture. *Diabetologia* 2004;47:1343–1353

9. Reiber GE, Vileikyte L, Boyko EJ, et al. Causal pathways for incident lower-extremity ulcers in patients with diabetes from two settings. *Diabetes Care* 1999;22:157–162

10. Lavery LA, Higgins KR, Lanctot DR, et al. Preventing diabetic foot ulcer recurrence in high-risk patients: use of temperature monitoring as a self-assessment tool. *Diabetes Care* 2007;30:14–20

Suggested Readings

Boulton AJM. The diabetic foot: preface. *Med Clin N Am* 2013;97:xiii–xiv

Boulton AJM, Cavanagh PR, Rayman G (Eds.). *The Foot in Diabetes.* 4th ed. Chichester, U.K., Wiley, 2006

Boulton AJM, Kirsner RS, Vileikyte L. Neuropathic diabetic foot ulcers. *N Engl J Med* 2004;351:48–55

Bowker JH, Pfeifer MA (Eds.). *Levin & O'Neal's The Diabetic Foot.* 7th ed. Philadelphia, Mosby Elsevier, 2008

Brem H, Sheehan P, Boulton AJ. Protocol for treatment of diabetic foot ulcers. *Am J Surg* 2004;187(Suppl. 5a):1S–10S

Jeffcoate WJ, Harding KG. Diabetic foot ulcers. *Lancet* 2003;361:1545–1551

Van Houtum WH, Boulton AJM (Eds.). The diabetic foot: proceedings of the 5th International Symposium on the Diabetic Foot. *Diabet Metab Res Rev* 24 2008;(Suppl.):S1–S202

2
The Comprehensive Diabetic Foot Examination and Risk Assessment

Andrew J.M. Boulton, MD, DSc (Hon), FRCP
Manchester Royal Infirmary, Division of Medicine, Manchester, U.K.

The comprehensive diabetic foot examination is essential to preventing ulcers and amputation. A task force of the American Diabetes Association (ADA) met early in 2008 to address and concisely summarize recent literature in the area and recommend what should be included in the comprehensive foot exam for adult patients with diabetes. Panel members of this committee, in addition to representing diabetes, were drawn from areas including primary care, orthopedic and vascular surgery, physical therapy, podiatric medicine and surgery, and the American Association for Clinical Endocrinologists. This chapter is a summary of the full report that was published in *Diabetes Care* in 2008.[1] Before the publication of this recent report, the ADA issued a position statement on preventive foot care in diabetes in 2003.[2]

The Pathway to Foot Ulceration

The pathway to foot ulceration is summarized in the previous chapter, where it is stated that a number of component causes, most important of which is peripheral neuropathy, interact to complete the causal pathway to foot ulceration. A list of the principal contributory factors that might result in foot ulcer development is provided in Table 2.1. Because identification of these patients at risk of foot problems is the first step in preventing such complications, this chapter will focus on key components of the foot examination.

DOI: 10.2337/9781580405706.02

Table 2.1 Risk Factors for Foot Ulcers

Previous amputation
Past foot ulcer history
Peripheral neuropathy
Foot deformity
Peripheral vascular disease
Visual impairment
Diabetic nephropathy (especially patients on dialysis)
Poor glycemic control
Cigarette smoking

Reprinted with permission from Boulton et al.[1]

Components of the Foot Exam

History

Although history is always a pivotal component of risk assessment, since up to 50% of patients at risk of foot problems will have no symptoms whatsoever, the patient cannot be fully assessed for risk factors based on history alone. A careful foot exam remains the essential component of this process.

Key components of the history include a past history of ulceration or amputation and other important assessments, including the history of neuropathic or vascular symptoms, which are listed in Table 2.2. Because it is increasingly recognized that foot ulcers are extremely common in patients undergoing renal replacement therapy (dialysis) or post-transplant, renal replacement therapy or transplants are key components of the history.[3,4]

General Inspection

After patients have removed their shoes and socks, a careful examination of the feet in a well-lit room should always be carried out. A quick inspection of footwear and foot deformities is indicated, and the question "Are these shoes appropriate for these feet?" should be asked. Features that should be assessed during the foot inspection are outlined in Table 2.3. One important and often overlooked or misdiagnosed condition is Charcot neuroarthropathy. Charcot neuroarthropathy occurs in the neuropathic foot and most often affects the mid-foot region. This condition may present acutely as a unilateral red, hot, and swollen foot with no obvious deformity, but in its later stages, flat foot

Table 2.2 Essential Features of History	
Past history	**Vascular symptoms**
• Ulceration	• Claudication
• Amputation	• Rest pain
• Charcot joint	• Nonhealing ulcer
• Vascular surgery	
• Angioplasty	**Other diabetes complications**
• Cigarette smoking	• Renal (dialysis, transplant)
	• Retinal (visual impairment)
Neuropathic symptoms	
• Positive (e.g., burning or shooting pain, electrical or sharp sensations)	
• Negative (e.g., numbness, feet feel dead)	

Reprinted with permission from Boulton et al.[1]

with profound deformities may be present. Any patient with suspect Charcot neuroarthropathy should be immediately referred to a foot specialist for further assessment and care.

Neurological Assessment

As noted above, peripheral neuropathy is the most common component cause on the pathway to diabetic foot ulceration. The clinical examination recommended, however, is designed not to identify early neuropathy but to identify a loss of protective sensation due to neuropathy (LOPS). The diagnosis and management of neuropathy in general were covered in a 2004 ADA technical review.[5]

Five simple clinical tests (Table 2.3), each with evidence from well-conducted prospective clinical cohort studies, are considered useful in the diagnosis of LOPS in the diabetic foot.[1,2] The ADA task force agreed that any of the five tests listed could be used by clinicians to identify LOPS, although, ideally, two of these tests should be regularly performed during the screening exam: normally this would comprise the 10-g monofilament plus one other test. One or more abnormal tests would suggest LOPS, whereas at least two normal tests (and no abnormal test) would rule out LOPS. The last test listed, vibration assessment, using a biothesiometer or similar instrument, is widely used in the United States and Europe; however, identification of the patient with LOPS can easily be carried out without this or any other expensive electrical equipment.

Table 2.3 Key Components of the Diabetic Foot Exam

Inspection
- Dermatologic
  - Skin status: color, thickness, dryness, cracking
  - Sweating
  - Infection: check between toes for fungal infection
  - Ulceration
  - Calluses/blistering: hemorrhage into callus?
- Musculoskeletal
  - Deformity, e.g., claw toes, hammer toes, prominent metatarsal heads, Charcot joint
  - Muscle wasting (guttering between metatarsals)
- Neurological assessment
  - 10-g monofilament + one of the following[4]
  - Vibration using 128-Hz tuning fork
  - Pinprick sensation
  - Ankle reflexes
  - Vascular perception threshold
- Vascular assessment
  - Foot pulses
  - ABI, if indicated

Reprinted with permission from Boulton et al.[1]

- **10-g monofilaments.** Monofilaments, sometimes known as Semmes-Weinstein monofilaments, were used to diagnose sensory loss in leprosy.[6] However, many prospective studies have confirmed that loss of pressure sensation using the 10-g monofilament is highly predictive of subsequent ulceration. Screening for sensory loss with the 10-g monofilament is in widespread use across the United States, and its efficacy in this regard has been confirmed in a number of trials, including most recently the Seattle Diabetic Foot Study.[7]

  Monofilaments are constructed to buckle when a 10-g force is applied; loss of the ability to detect this pressure in one or more anatomical sites on the plantar surface of the foot has been associated with loss of large-fiber nerve function.

  It is recommended that four sites (first, third, and fifth metatarsal heads and the plantar surface of the distal hallux) be tested on each foot. Details of the technique for testing pressure perception with a

10-g monofilament are provided in the task force report.[1] Caution is indicated when selecting the brand of monofilament to use in clinical practice, as many commercially available monofilaments have been shown to be inaccurate.[8] Areas of callus should also be avoided when testing for pressure perception.

- **128-Hz tuning fork.** The tuning fork is widely used in clinical practice and provides an easy and inexpensive test of vibratory sensation. Vibration should be tested over the tip of the hallux bilaterally. An abnormal response can be defined as when the patient loses vibratory sensation, and the examiner still perceives it while holding the fork on the tip of the toe.

- **Pinprick sensation.** Similarly, the inability of the subject to perceive pinprick sensation has been associated with an increased risk of ulceration. A disposable pin should be applied just proximal to the toenail of the hallux, with just enough pressure to deform the skin. Inability to perceive pinprick over either hallux would be regarded as an abnormal result.

- **Ankle reflexes.** Absence of the ankle reflexes is associated with an increased risk of ulceration. Ankle reflexes can be tested with a patient either kneeling or resting on a couch/table. The Achilles tendon should be stretched until the ankle is in a neutral position before striking it with the tendon hammer. If a response is initially absent, the patient could be asked to hook the fingers together and pull, with the ankle reflexes then retested with this reinforcement. Total absence of the ankle reflex either at rest or upon reinforcement is regarded as an abnormal result.

- **Vibration perception threshold testing.** The biothesiometer (or neurothesiometer or vibration perception threshold [VPT] meter) is a simple handheld device that gives semiquantitative assessment of VPT. As for the 128-Hz tuning fork, vibration perception using the biothesiometer is also tested over the pulp of the hallux. A VPT reading of >25 V is regarded as abnormal and has been shown to be strongly predictive of subsequent foot ulceration.[9]

Vascular Assessment

Peripheral arterial disease is a component cause in approximately one-third to one-half of all foot ulcers and is often a significant risk factor associated with recurrent wounds. The assessment of peripheral arterial disease (PAD) is therefore of vital importance in the annual foot exam. The vascular examination should include palpation of the posterior tibial and dorsalis pedis pulses,[10] which should be characterized as either "present" or "absent."

Those patients with signs or symptoms of vascular disease (Table 2.2) or abnormal pulses on screening should undergo an ankle-brachial pressure index (ABI) and be considered for possible referral to a vascular specialist. The ABI is a simple and easily reproducible method of diagnosing vascular insufficiency in the lower limbs. The technique is outlined in the task force report.[1] However, it must be remembered that vascular calcification is common in patients at risk of foot problems and may give rise to false elevation of the ABI. Although the ADA consensus panel on PAD recommended measurement of the ABI in diabetic patients over 50 years of age on an annual basis,[11] it is recognized that this might not be possible in many instances in primary care.

Risk Classification and Referral/Follow-Up

Once patients have been thoroughly assessed as described above, they should be assigned to a foot risk category (Table 2.4). These categories are designed to direct referral and subsequent therapy by the clinician or team[12] and frequency of follow-up by the generalist or specialist. An increase in category assignment is associated with increased ulceration, hospitalization, and even amputation. Patients in risk category 0 do not need referral and should receive a general foot care education and undergo a comprehensive diabetic foot examination on an annual basis. Patients in the other categories should be managed as outlined in Table 2.4.

Conclusions

It cannot be overemphasized that diabetic foot complications are common, complex, and costly, and they mandate aggressive and proactive preventive assessments by generalists and specialists. All patients with diabetes must have their feet evaluated at least annually for the presence of predisposing factors for ulceration and amputation. This chapter has summarized the simple protocol for doing just that. If abnormalities are found on examination, more frequent evaluation of the diabetic foot is recommended, depending on the risk category, as outlined in Table 2.4.

Table 2.4 Risk Classification Based on the Comprehensive Foot Examination

Risk Category	Definition	Treatment Recommendations	Suggested Follow-Up
0	No LOPS, no PAD, no deformity	• Patient education including advice on appropriate footwear	Annually (by generalist and/or specialist)
1	LOPS ± deformity	• Consider prescriptive or accommodative footwear • Consider prophylactic surgery if deformity is not able to be safely accommodated in shoes; continue patient education	Every 3–6 months (by generalist or specialist)
2	PAD ± LOPS	• Consider prescriptive or accommodative footwear • Consider vascular consultation for combined follow-up	Every 2–3 months (by specialist)
3	History of ulcer or amputation	• Same as category 1 • Consider vascular consultation for combined follow-up if PAD present	Every 1–2 months (by specialist)

Reprinted with permission from Boulton et al.[1]

References

1. Boulton AJM, Armstrong DG, Albert SF, et al. Comprehensive foot examination and risk assessment: a report of the Task Force of the Foot Care Interest Group of the American Diabetes Association, with endorsement by the American Association of Clinical Endocrinologists. *Diabetes Care* 2008;31:1679–1685

2. American Diabetes Association. Preventive foot care in people with diabetes. *Diabetes Care* 2003;26(Suppl. 1):S78–S79

3. Game FL, Chipchase SY, Hubbart R, Burden RP, Jeffcoate WJ. Temporal association between the incidence of foot ulceration and the start of dialysis in diabetes mellitus. *Nephrol Dialysis Transplant* 2006;21:3207–3210

4. Ndip A, Lavery LA, La Fontaine J, et al. High levels of foot ulceration and amputation risk in a multiracial cohort of diabetic patients on dialysis therapy. *Diabetes Care* 2010;33:878–880

5. Boulton AJM, Malik RA, Arezzo JC, Sosenko JM. Diabetic somatic neuropathy. *Diabetes Care* 2004;27:1458–1486

6. Mayfield JA, Sugerman JR. The use of the Semmes-Weinstein monofilament and other threshold tests for preventing foot ulceration and amputation in persons with diabetes. *J Fam Pract* 2000;49(Suppl. 11):S17–S29

7. Boyko EJ, Ahroni JH, Cohen V, Nelson KM, Heagerty PJ. Prediction of diabetic foot ulcer occurrence using commonly available clinical information: the Seattle Diabetic Foot Study. *Diabetes Care* 2006;29:1202–1207

8. Booth J, Young MJ. Differences in the performance of commercially available 10-g monofilaments. *Diabetes Care* 2000;23:984–988

9. Abbott CA, Vileikyte L, Williamson S, Carrington AL, Boulton AJM. Multicentre study of the incidence of and predictive risk factors for diabetic neuropathic foot ulceration. *Diabetes Care* 1998;21:1071–1075

10. Khan NA, Rahim SA, Anand SS, Simel DL, Panju A. Does the clinical examination predict lower extremity peripheral arterial disease? *JAMA* 2006;295:536–546

11. American Diabetes Association. Peripheral arterial disease in people with diabetes. *Diabetes Care* 2003;26:3333–3341

12. Lavery LA, Peters EJ, Williams JR, et al. Re-evaluating how we classify the diabetic foot: restructuring the diabetic foot risk classification system of the International Working Group on the Diabetic Foot. *Diabetes Care* 2008;31:154–156

3
Shoes and Insoles for At-Risk People with Diabetes

Jan S. Ulbrecht, MD,[1] and Peter R. Cavanagh, PhD, DSc[2]

[1]*Department of Medicine, Penn State University, University Park, PA, and*
[2]*Department of Orthopaedics, University of Washington College of Medicine, Seattle, WA*

In the United States, diabetes is the leading cause of nontraumatic lower-extremity amputation (60,000–70,000 cases per year[1]), and amputation is usually preceded by a foot ulcer. Among Medicare beneficiaries, 8.1% had a foot ulcer in 2007,[2] and in earlier studies, it was estimated that 15–25% of all people with diabetes will experience a foot ulcer at some point in their lifetime.[3] Footwear can both cause and prevent foot injury. Therefore, practitioners treating patients with diabetes must understand the principles and practice of comprehensive foot care, including the prescription of appropriate footwear. The clinician's evaluation of footwear and insoles should be a standard part of the lower-extremity examination in primary diabetes care.

Who Is at Risk for Foot Injury?

As discussed in more detail in Chapter 2, identification of patients at risk for foot injury who will benefit from enhanced self-care and therapeutic footwear begins with an assessment of sensation in the foot. If patients cannot feel the touch of a 10-g monofilament, they are said to have lost protective sensation and thus may injure their feet without knowing it. In patients with foot deformities (such as bunions, prominent metatarsal head[s], clawed or hammered toes, or a mid-foot prominence as a result of Charcot neuroarthropathy), injury may occur at the site of the deformity because of repetitive elevated plantar pressure during walking, or on the non-plantar surfaces because of poor footwear fit. Impaired lower-extremity circulation, indicated for example by a low ankle-brachial index,[1] is also a risk factor for foot injury. In addition, all patients with a prior ulcer should be considered at risk, as should patients with any foot amputation, including partial amputation of toes.

Although it seems intuitive that risk would be greater for individuals who are more active, because of the greater cumulative stress on the foot, available evidence (as reviewed, for example, in an article by Lemaster et al.[4]) does not support this point of view. Rather, it appears that people who are more active may have a lower risk of ulceration (perhaps through some form of tissue conditioning), *but* markedly higher activity above the background average may be a risk. Thus, high-risk patients should be encouraged to use a pedometer routinely to avoid walking in excess of their customary activity level, to be wary of high-activity days (e.g., travel, Christmas shopping at the mall), and to return to normal activity slowly and cautiously after a period of reduced activity, such as a hospitalization.

Evidence Base for Therapeutic Footwear

Footwear as a Cause of Injury

Considerable anecdotal evidence and opinion indicate that shoes can cause foot injury.[5–8] Various authors have suggested that 21–82% of foot ulcers are related to pressure from footwear that is too narrow or otherwise inadequate. These rates refer primarily to injuries to the non-plantar surface of the foot. In this context, it is noteworthy that many diabetic patients wear shoes that are too small.[9] In one study, 93% of U.S. veterans with loss of protective sensation (LOPS) were wearing shoes that were too small,[10] which is consistent with the hypothesis that patients with poor sensation prefer tighter shoes, so they can "feel" them better. This has important implications for patient care and education—knowledgeable professionals should fit shoes for high-risk patients, if possible, and, when not possible, patients must be taught the principles of selecting appropriate footwear and of a break-in for new shoes (see Other Footwear Issues in this chapter).

Footwear for Primary Prevention

Many foot ulcers occur on the plantar surface at points of high plantar pressure, most frequently under the metatarsal heads. Therapeutic footwear can distribute load and thus reduce pressure at these points and therefore should have utility in preventing such ulcers. No studies that examine the role of footwear in preventing the first ulcer in at-risk people with diabetes have yet appeared in the literature.[11] However, footwear does have a protective effect in secondary prevention, and prescribing appropriate footwear as primary prevention for all patients who have risk factors for foot injury is a prudent measure.

Footwear for Secondary Prevention

Ulcer recurrence is the dominant problem in treating diabetic foot disease. Estimates for annual recurrence vary from <5% to almost 60%,[12–16] depending on the level of care offered. The relative risk of an ulcer for patients with a history of prior ulcer is ~10 times that of patients without such history.[17] Extensive evidence suggests a protective effect of footwear to prevent ulcer recurrence, although much of this had, until recently, come from clinical studies that were not always randomized or appropriately controlled.[11,15] A large randomized controlled trial[18] showed that prescribed footwear was better than no prescription in preventing ulcers. While this is something that most clinicians will find obvious, there is at least evidence that now supports this basic tenet of foot care. Another randomized controlled study has shown that one clinician's design for a custom insole was not superior to an off-the-shelf product as far as plantar pressure reduction was concerned. Although limited in its generalizability, this study is important because it demonstrates that simply providing the patient with "a custom insole" is not a guarantee of improving the mechanical environment for the foot. However, there are now two randomized controlled trials[13,16] comparing the effect of footwear with enhanced offloading to control footwear with regard to ulcer prevention. These studies have now unequivocally clarified the protective effect of footwear that demonstrably offloads areas of high plantar pressure.

Footwear for Patients with Ulcers

Patients with foot ulcers should not wear shoes that they would use for normal day-to-day wear, because shoes of this type cannot, in general, provide the mechanical offloading needed to accomplish healing. Various approaches to offloading during healing are discussed in Chapter 5, including "healing shoes." These shoes are designed to provide temporary removal of pressure in either the forefoot or rearfoot.[11]

Practice

Goals of Footwear Intervention

Broadly speaking, "therapeutic footwear" must serve at least five goals. It should 1) provide sufficient room to accommodate a potentially deformed foot and an insole, 2) protect the plantar surface by reducing plantar pressure as appropriate (see below), 3) be functional in all the situations the patient faces, 4) be cosmetically adequate so that the patient will use it, and 5) be part of a solution in case the patient has problems with stability, which is common in patients with neuropathy.[19] These goals are not always congruent, and compromises must often be made. For instance, in general, the better the plantar offloading attributes of the shoe, the more it tends to impede stability. In addition, patient preference is often a dominant factor. The consequences of such compromises should be explained to the patient. Although the provider of diabetes care does not typically have the skills to design therapeutic footwear, he or she should nevertheless understand these goals as a basis for developing a relationship with a local footwear supplier to whom at-risk patients can be referred with confidence.

Choice of Footwear

Practitioners prescribing footwear for at-risk patients must consider the lifestyle of the patient. Typically, patients need footwear that is suited to their occupation, leisure activities, weather exposure, and home use, including footwear to avoid nighttime barefoot walking that might present a significant risk of ulceration. Achieving all this with the one pair of shoes per year that is usually covered by insurance is challenging, but it can be achieved by adding different types of footwear to the patient's inventory over several years. Another option is the use of rubber overshoes for inclement weather. Table 3.1 presents a guide to prescription footwear based on the patient's risk of foot injury.

Patients at the low end of the "at-risk" spectrum can frequently use wide, well-fitting athletic shoes without any modification. Such shoes can reduce plantar pressure by up to 30% and have been reported to reduce plantar callus.[20,21] Patients who need more protection should be fitted with "depth shoes,"

Table 3.1 General Guide to Footwear Prescription Based on Risk Status		
Plantar injury risk (in addition to LOPS or significant peripheral vascular disease)	Plantar support surface	Shoe/toe-box depth, etc.
None	Off-the-shelf sports shoe or depth shoe with a soft insole	Assure appropriate shoe depth, or modify shoe upper or use custom molded shoe to accommodate non-plantar deformity
Moderate (prominent plantar callus, occasionally hemorrhagic)	Depth shoe with a thick custom-molded insole; consider additional customizations such as metatarsal pad, bar, relief	
Severe (recurring plantar ulcer or hemorrhagic callus or major surgical deformity)	Depth shoe with a thick custom molded insole plus customizations such metatarsal pad, bar, relief; consider rocker outsole; consider referral to a specialized center that uses measured plantar pressure in footwear design^	

^Benefit demonstrated by Bus et al.[13] and Ulbrecht et al.[16]

which provide enough height in the forefoot area to allow for a thick insole (flat or customized; see Choice of Insoles below) without forcing the dorsum of the foot up against the shoe upper.

To accommodate foot deformity, a qualified pedorthist (a practitioner who is certified by the Pedorthic Footwear Association; http://www.pedorthics.org) can make custom shoes over models of the patient's feet, although stretching the shoe uppers with special tools can accommodate some lesser deformities.

Finally, some individuals with weakness or instability at the joints of the foot or ankle may need wedges or flares built into the shoe or braces that can improve stability and/or transfer some load from the foot to the leg.

Choice of Insoles

The main purpose of the insoles in footwear for at-risk diabetic patients is the reduction of plantar pressure under high-risk regions, such as the metatarsal heads, rigid big toes, or the tips of deformed lesser toes. Thus, insoles for patients with LOPS should accommodate rather than "correct." Functional orthotics, the in-shoe devices that are widely used to correct foot alignment (in sports medicine, for example), tend to increase loading and are therefore typically not appropriate for neuropathic patients.

The stock insoles delivered with most therapeutic shoes are "fillers" and need to be replaced before the patient can wear the shoes. As noted above, the insoles in sports shoes may be sufficient for some patients. Flat insoles of sufficient thickness can deliver significant offloading,[22] and patients with high-risk feet should use insoles of up to 3/8 of an inch if there is room in the shoe. Recent studies have shown a difference between pressure relief of insoles after 6 and 12 months of use compared to the new condition, but not between 6 and 12 months. This suggests that most compression occurs in the first 6 months and may be a reason for changing insoles more frequently.

Beyond thickness, insoles can be customized with specifically placed "reliefs" or supports (the best known are metatarsal pads or bars) that transfer load to other regions of the foot.[23,24] Pedorthists and orthotists are skilled in making such modifications, but recent studies have shown that such modifications should be made with measurement of plantar pressure whenever possible, particularly for patients who are reulcerating.[13,16]

Patients should be given several pairs of insoles when shoes are dispensed, so that they can be used in rotation, to reduce insole wear. Thick socks (similar to sport socks) are also effective in reducing pressure,[25] but they must be used only when there is sufficient room in the shoes.

For patients at very high risk of plantar injury, shoes may be modified to have rigid "rocker" or "roller" outsoles that, along with an appropriate insole, allow patients to walk without significantly extending their toes at the metatarso-phalangeal joints. This design has been shown to reduce plantar pressure by as much as 50%.[26] Patients who are prescribed rocker or roller shoes may initially complain of instability, and they should be advised to use their shoes for progressively longer periods until they feel more secure.

The Footwear Prescription

The following steps provide a useful approach to the therapeutic footwear prescription:

1. Determine the intended use of the shoe—e.g., home, work, waterproof, all-weather outsole.
2. Select the level of plantar protection required—thickness of insole, reliefs and supports, rocker bottom.
3. Decide the volume/shape of the shoe needed to accommodate dorsal deformity and the insole selected—sports shoe, depth shoe, stretches and reliefs of the upper, custom-molded upper.
4. Address stability issues—outsole flares, wedges, bracing, aids to walking.

This same framework should be used in the primary care office to assess adequacy of the footwear an at-risk patient owns and wears.

Medicare Guidelines

For the patient to be eligible for the Medicare diabetic therapeutic footwear benefit, the treating physician must provide a written statement certifying that at least one of the following conditions exists:

- History of partial or complete amputation of the foot
- History of previous foot ulceration
- History of pre-ulcerative calluses
- Peripheral neuropathy with evidence of callus formation
- Foot deformity
- Poor circulation

Coverage in one calendar year is provided for one pair of custom-molded footwear plus two pairs of insoles, or one pair of extra-depth footwear and three pairs of insoles. Shoe modifications (such as wedges, flares, roller/rocker, metatarsal bars) may be substituted for a pair of insoles. The footwear must meet the Medicare definitions of depth for custom-molded shoes. Many other insurance plans follow the same criteria.

Other Footwear Issues

As is apparent from this discussion, there is no such thing as a "diabetic shoe," only an appropriate shoe for any given at-risk patient, and for some, this can be a simple sports shoe. Conversely, just because the shoe is special and/or expensive does not guarantee that it is right for any given at-risk patient at a given time.

Furthermore, the best prescription footwear is not effective if patients do not use it,[13] and footwear use by patients, particularly in the home, is often quite low.[27] Thus, clinicians must work with their patients to help them optimally use appropriate footwear, once such footwear has been prescribed and dispensed. Patients must understand that wearing the prescribed shoes falls into the same category as taking medication—something that is essential for preserving their health. A technique such as Motivational Interviewing, an approach to interacting with patients that is rapidly entering primary care, may be helpful.[28] A high-risk patient by virtue of LOPS should have his or her feet examined at each primary care visit, which provides an opportunity to reinforce footwear use in the primary care setting. In some cases, it may be necessary to "go home with the patient." This would entail exploring footwear use from the moment the person wakes up, all the way through the next night, including trips to the bathroom. For some patients, even barefoot trips to the bathroom or standing barefoot in the shower, while using prescribed footwear for all other weight-bearing activity, is enough to cause ulceration. Beware of the patient who responds to a question about barefoot walking with an emphatic "no." Further probing sometimes reveals that the person routinely walks at home in socks only. Providing patients with a second pair of appropriate shoes for home use may be important,[16,27] but no studies have as yet directly examined this issue.

Another important aspect of providing footwear to at-risk patients is the "prescription" of a break-in protocol. Those of us with sensate feet are guided by discomfort to wear new shoes often just an hour or two the first day, to avoid blisters; after a few days, the leather upper "breaks in," causing no further problems. While there have been no specific studies of this practice, the process is usually to give a person with LOPS a specific break-in schedule, for instance, recommending use of new footwear for an hour in the morning and an hour in the afternoon the first day and increasing by an hour every day.

The syndrome of the "holiday ulcer" is commonplace[29]: many ulcers develop at weddings, funerals, or religious events or on vacation because the patient selects inappropriate footwear "just this once" and usually engages in increased activity. Asking patients as part of the foot examination about upcoming special events may prevent problems.

In summary, success of therapeutic footwear is in part a function of patient behavior and in part a function of footwear design. Recent developments in both areas suggest that improvements in outcomes should be expected. Historically, footwear feature selection/design had often been a trial-and-error process in which success was not assured, and where lack of success meant another ulcer. At this point, the foundation has been laid for designing more effective shoes using measurement, particularly plantar pressure measurement,[13,16] and these findings await widespread translation into routine care.

Conflict of Interest

Both authors own stock in DIApedia LLC and are inventors on U.S. patents 6 610 897, 6 720 470, and 7 206 718, which elucidate a load-relieving dressing and a method of insole manufacture for offloading diabetic feet.

References

1. Centers for Disease Control and Prevention. http://www.cdc.gov/diabetes/statistics/complications_national.htm. Accessed October 2014

2. Margolis DJ, Gupta J, Hoffstad O, et al. Lack of effectiveness of hyperbaric oxygen therapy for the treatment of diabetic foot ulcer and the prevention of amputation: a cohort study. *Diabetes Care* 2013;36:1961–1966

3. Singh N, Armstrong DG, Lipsky BA. Preventing foot ulcers in patients with diabetes. *JAMA* 2005;293:217–228

4. Lemaster JW, Mueller MJ, Reiber GE, et al. Effect of weight-bearing activity on foot ulcer incidence in people with diabetic peripheral neuropathy: feet first randomized controlled trial. *Phys Ther* 2008;88:1385–1398

5. Edmonds ME, Blundell MP, Morris ME, et al. Improved survival of the diabetic foot: the role of a specialized foot clinic. *Q J Med* 1986; 60:763–771

6. Apelqvist J, Larsson J, Agardh CD. The influence of external precipitating factors and peripheral neuropathy on the development and outcome of diabetic foot ulcers. *J Diabetes Complications* 1990;4:21–25

7. Reiber GE. Who is at risk of limb loss and what to do about it? *J Rehabil Res Dev* 1994;31:357–362

8. Macfarlane RM, Jeffcoate WJ. Factors contributing to the presentation of diabetic foot ulcers. *Diabet Med* 1997;14:867–870

9. Harrison SJ, Cochrane L, Abboud RJ, Leese GP. Do patients with diabetes wear shoes of the correct size? *Int J Clin Pract* 2007;61:1900–1904

10. Nixon BP, Armstrong DG, Wendell C, et al. Do US veterans wear appropriately sized shoes? The Veterans Affairs shoe size selection study. *J Am Podiatr Med Assoc* 2006;96:290–292

11. Bus SA, Valk GD, van Deursen RW, et al. The effectiveness of footwear and offloading interventions to prevent and heal foot ulcers and reduce plantar pressure in diabetes: a systematic review. *Diabetes Metab Res Rev* 2008;24(Suppl. 1):S162–S180

12. Armstrong DG, Holtz-Neiderer K, Wendel C, et al. Skin temperature monitoring reduces the risk for diabetic foot ulceration in high-risk patients. *Am J Med* 2007;120:1042–1046

13. Bus SA, Waaijman R, Arts M, et al. Effect of custom-made footwear on foot ulcer recurrence in diabetes: a multicenter randomized controlled trial. *Diabetes Care* 2013;36:4109–4116

14. Lavery LA, Higgins KR, Lanctot DR, et al. Preventing diabetic foot ulcer recurrence in high-risk patients: use of temperature monitoring as a self-assessment tool. *Diabetes Care* 2007;30:14–20

15. Maciejewski ML, Reiber GE, Smith DG, et al. Effectiveness of diabetic therapeutic footwear in preventing reulceration. *Diabetes Care* 2004;27:1774–1782

16. Ulbrecht JS, Hurley T, Mauger DT, Cavanagh PR. Prevention of recurrent foot ulcers with plantar pressure-based in-shoe orthoses: the CareFUL Prevention Multicenter Randomized Controlled Trial. *Diabetes Care* 2014;37:1982–1989

17. Abbott CA, Carrington AL, Ashe H, et al. The North-West Diabetes Foot Care Study: incidence of, and risk factors for, new diabetic foot ulceration in a community-based patient cohort. *Diabet Med* 2002;19:377–384

18. Rizzo L, Tedeschi A, Fallani E, et al. Custom-made orthoses and shoes in a structured follow-up program reduces the incidence of neuropathic ulcers in high-risk diabetic foot patients. *Int J Low Extrem Wounds* 2012;11:59–64

19. Bonnet C, Carello C, Turvey MT. Diabetes and postural stability: review and hypotheses. *J Mot Behav* 2009;41:172–190

20. Perry JE, Ulbrecht JS, Derr JA, Cavanagh PR. The use of running shoes to reduce plantar pressures in patients who have diabetes. *J Bone Joint Surg Am* 1995;77:1819–1828

21. Soulier SM. The use of running shoes in the prevention of plantar diabetic ulcers. *J Am Podiatr Med Assoc* 1986;76:395–400

22. Rogers K, Otter SJ, Birch I. The effect of PORON and Plastazote insoles on forefoot plantar pressures. *British Journal of Podiatry* 2006;9:111–114

23. Mueller MJ, Lott DJ, Hastings MK, et al. Efficacy and mechanism of orthotic devices to unload metatarsal heads in people with diabetes and a history of plantar ulcers. *Phys Ther* 2006;86:833–842

24. Guldemond NA, Leffers P, Schaper NC, et al. The effects of insole configurations on forefoot plantar pressure and walking convenience in diabetic patients with neuropathic feet. *Clin Biomech (Bristol, Avon)* 2007;22:81–87.

25. Veves A, Masson EA, Fernando DJ, Boulton AJ. Use of experimental padded hosiery to reduce abnormal foot pressures in diabetic neuropathy. *Diabetes Care* 1989;12:653–655

26. van Schie C, Ulbrecht JS, Becker MB, Cavanagh PR. Design criteria for rigid rocker shoes. *Foot Ankle Int* 2000;21:833–844

27. Waaijman R, Keukenkamp R, de Haart M, et al. Adherence to wearing prescription custom-made footwear in patients with diabetes at high risk for plantar foot ulceration. *Diabetes Care* 2013;36:1613–1618

28. Gabbay RA, Kaul S, Ulbrecht J, Scheffler NM, Armstrong DG. Motivational interviewing by podiatric physicians: a method for improving patient self-care of the diabetic foot. *J Am Podiatr Med Assoc* 2011;101:78–84

29. Armstrong DG, Dang C, Nixon BP, Boulton AJ. The hazards of the holiday foot: persons at high risk for diabetic foot ulceration may be more active on holiday. *Diabet Med* 2007;20:247–248

Suggested Readings

Boulton AJ, Armstrong DG, Albert SF, et al. Comprehensive foot examination and risk assessment: a report of the task force of the foot care interest group of the American Diabetes Association, with endorsement by the American Association of Clinical Endocrinologists. *Diabetes Care* 2008;31:1679–1685

Foto JG, Birke JA. Evaluation of multidensity orthotic materials used in footwear for patients with diabetes. *Foot Ankle Int* 1998;19:836–841

Owings TM, Woerner JL, Frampton JD, et al. Custom therapeutic insoles based on both foot shape and plantar pressure measurement provide enhanced pressure relief. *Diabetes Care* 2008;31:839–844

Paton JS, Stenhouse EA, Bruce G, et al. A comparison of customised and prefabricated insoles to reduce risk factors for neuropathic diabetic foot ulceration: a participant-blinded randomised controlled trial. *J Foot Ankle Res.* 2012;5:31

Paton JS, Stenhouse E, Bruce G, Jones R. A longitudinal investigation into the functional and physical durability of insoles used for the preventive management of neuropathic diabetic feet. *J Am Podiatr Med Assoc* 2014;104:50–57

Reiber GE, Smith DG, Wallace C, et al. Effect of therapeutic footwear on foot reulceration in patients with diabetes: a randomized controlled trial. *JAMA* 2002;287:2552–2558

Sargen MR, Hoffstad O, Margolis DJ. Geographic variation in Medicare spending and mortality for diabetic patients with foot ulcers and amputations. *J Diabetes Complications* 2013;27:128–133.

Wooldridge J, Bergeron J, Thornton C. Preventing diabetic foot disease: lessons from the Medicare therapeutic shoe demonstration. *Am J Public Health* 1996;86:935–938

4
Ulcer Assessment and Classification

Nicolaas C. Schaper, MD
Division of Endocrinology, University of Maastricht, Maastricht, the Netherlands

In diabetic patients, the foot is the crossroads of several pathological processes. Almost all components of the lower extremity are involved: skin, subcutaneous tissue, muscles, bones, joints, blood vessels, and nerves.[1] Because each of these components can contribute to foot ulcers, a multidisciplinary approach is needed, and a standardized assessment is essential to guide further diagnostic workup and therapy. In the past decade, much knowledge was obtained on the different underlying pathologies determining the outcome of an individual ulcer. If assessed in a standardized way, the prognosis of the ulcer and the limb can be estimated, and the urgency of specific interventions can be determined to limit further tissue loss (time = tissue). A diabetic foot ulcer is here defined as any "full-thickness" lesion of the skin—that is, a wound penetrating through the dermis. Lesions such as blisters or skin mycosis are not defined as ulcers.[1]

Standardized Assessment

One of the pitfalls in assessing a foot ulcer is the limited value of history-taking. If patients have loss of sensation, limited mobility, and poor vision, they may not even be aware that they have a foot ulcer. In addition, both patient and clinician can be mistakenly reassured by the paucity of ulcer symptoms. However, the absence of symptoms generally does not rule out infection or critical limb

DOI: 10.2337/9781580405706.04

ischemia, and the other way around symptoms such as fever or pain frequently suggest severe problems, necessitating extensive evaluation.

Perfusion (Ischemia and Critical Limb Ischemia)

Several large-scale studies show that peripheral arterial disease (PAD) is present in up to 50% of all patients and that it is a major factor affecting wound healing. Therefore, the first goal in vascular examination is to exclude PAD with reasonable certainty in all patients. Claudication and ischemic rest pain are absent in many ischemic foot ulcers, probably because of sensory neuropathy, but if they are present, the risk of amputation is greatly enhanced, and an aggressive vascular evaluation should be performed. Additional signs of (severe) ischemia are multiple sites of skin necrosis, gangrene, and blanching of the feet when they are elevated, with a red-purple discoloration when the patient is standing or when the leg is in dependency. Please note that the feet can be red and relatively warm despite severe ischemia, probably because of the relative high shunt blood flow, a consequence of autonomic neuropathy.

In all patients, the proximal vessels, particularly the iliofemoral segment, should be auscultated for bruits. The pulses of the femoral, popliteal, dorsalis pedis, and posterior tibial artery should be palpated. Unfortunately, palpation of foot pulses is not always reliable, and patients with palpable pulses can still have severe PAD.[2,3] Therefore, because simple screening tests the flow, signals from both foot arteries should be evaluated with a handheld Doppler, and the ankle brachial index (ABI) should be measured.

PAD is unlikely if:

- The patients has no symptoms (claudication/rest pain) *and*
- Bi- or triphasic signals are heard with handheld Doppler *and*
- The ABI is between 0.9 and 1.3.

However, the lower leg arteries can become less compressible because of media calcification, resulting in falsely elevated Doppler ankle pressures in up to one-third of all patients. Systolic toe pressures and transcutaneous oxygen pressure ($TcPo_2$) can provide additional information in these patients. Both a toe-brachial index <0.7 in a foot acclimatized in a warm surrounding and a $TcPo_2$ <50–60 mmHg in a foot without severe edema strongly suggest PAD.[2]

Once the diagnosis of PAD is made, its severity (i.e., its effect on wound healing) should be assessed. Systolic toe pressures and $TcPo_2$ probably predict wound healing more reliably than the ABI. Prediction of wound healing based on perfusion testing, regardless of method, follows a sigmoid curve. Most ulcers can heal if the toe pressure is >55 mmHg and the $TcPo_2$ >50 mmHg. Lower values are associated with a higher risk of poor healing and amputation, but no precise cutoff values can be given, since the effect of PAD on wound healing greatly depends on both local wound and patient characteristics. For instance, a relatively mild perfusion defect can have only limited effects on healing of a minor superficial ulcer, but can be sufficient to prevent wound healing in the case of an infected foot ulcer with chronic osteomyelitis. Therefore, if clinical and/or noninvasive assessments suggest PAD, a vascular surgeon should be consulted and revascularization considered.

In general, healing is usually severely impaired when[3]:

- The ABI is <0.6 *or*
- The toe pressure is <30 mmHg *or*
- The $TcPo_2$ is <30 mmHg.

Microvascular abnormalities do not play a major role in the pathogenesis of diabetic foot ulcers, and microangiopathy is no excuse for poorly healing wounds. If the wound has no healing tendency in 3–6 weeks despite optimal therapy, PAD should always be considered and further evaluation should be performed, despite the absence of abnormalities on initial testing.

Location, Depth, and Size

The location of an ulcer can give clues to its cause and will help to determine whether and how pressure relief should be applied. Neuropathic ulcers are usually located on areas with elevated pressure, such as the plantar side of the foot; ischemic or neuroischemic ulcers are more common on the tips of the toes or the lateral border. Because the ulcer is frequently covered by callus or necrotic tissue, the extent of tissue loss should be evaluated after initial debridement, but this should be performed judiciously when severe limb ischemia is suspected. Because of neuropathy, anesthesia is usually not necessary. In clinical practice, ulcers can be divided into two types: lesions confined to the skin (superficial) and ulcers with tissue loss or infection deeper than the skin (deep).[1] Heel ulcers and deep ulcers are associated with a poorer outcome. Ulcer size is easily estimated by multiplying the largest diameter by the second largest diameter measured perpendicular to the first diameter.

Infection

Infection of the diabetic foot is one of the major reasons for lower-extremity amputation. In particular, the combination of infection and PAD has a poor prognosis, and this combination should be considered a medical emergency (a "foot attack"). Unfortunately, no gold standard exists for diagnosing an infection, and signs can be subtle, despite extensive tissue destruction. A superficial infection (not extending through the fascia) without systemic signs can be diagnosed based on local swelling, purulent discharge, erythema, foul smell, or local tenderness or pain. A swab of the surface of the ulcer is of little value for microbiological diagnosis because the ulcer is usually colonized by various microorganisms.[4] Preferably, pus or a curettement of the ulcer base is obtained after debridement. Fever or laboratory signs of inflammation are frequently absent in patients with a deep abscess, but if present, even in patients with relative minor abnormalities on clinical examination, the foot should be extensively evaluated for a deep infection.

Osteomyelitis can also pose diagnostic problems. With an infected ulcer, if bone is explored with a metal probe before debridement, the risk of osteomyelitis is increased. An X-ray should be considered for any infected ulcer, but it may take several weeks before radiological changes appear, and a normal X-ray does not exclude osteomyelitis. A repeat X-ray after 2–4 weeks can be helpful, but X-rays are not very specific. Bone scans are more sensitive, but again, specificity is relatively low. MRIs are currently considered the most accurate imaging technique.[4] A more definitive diagnosis and reliable isolation of the causative microorganism(s) can be obtained with a bone biopsy.

Sensation, Biomechanical Evaluation, and Immediate Cause

Polyneuropathy is a major factor in foot ulceration, resulting in loss of protective sensation, muscle paralysis with subsequent deformities, abnormal walking patterns, and abnormal loading of the foot. The Semmes-Weinstein monofilament is a simple tool to assess loss of sensation. This inexpensive instrument consists of a fiber that buckles at a standardized pressure force, usually 10 g when examining for loss of protective sensation due to neuropathy (LOPS). Place the monofilament perpendicular to the surface of the skin, as described in Chapter 2. Vibration perception, determined with a 128-Hz tuning fork at the hallux, is an additional simple test.[1]

Callus and foot deformities—such as hallux valgus, prominent metatarsal heads, or hammering or clawing of the toes—are easily recognized during inspection of the feet, which should be performed with the patient both supine and standing. Abnormalities near an ulcer suggest increased biomechanical stress as a direct cause. Mobility in the first toe (hallux rigidus) and in the ankle joint should be estimated in plantar ulcerations, but these measurements are difficult to standardize. Finally, examine both of the shoes and socks. The fit of the footwear is especially important to evaluate, since most diabetic foot ulcers are caused by poorly fitting shoes and insoles.

Classification

Various systems have been proposed to classify diabetic foot ulcers, such as the Meggitt-Wagner system, the University of Texas system, and the S(AD) SAD system [Size (Area Depth) Sepsis Arteriopathy Denervation] (Table 4.1). Unfortunately, none has gained universal acceptance.[5-7] The University of Texas system is a validated extension of the well-known Wagner system and includes such vital items as depth and the presence of ischemia or infection; it also gives information about the risk of amputation from an individual ulcer.[6] One of the attractions of this system is that it underlines the poor prognosis of the combination of ischemia and infection. The PEDIS (Perfusion, Extent, Depth, Infection, Sensation) system was recently developed by an international consensus group for research purposes; this system, which was used in this chapter, gives criteria for several abnormalities.[8] The most simple scheme describing an ulcer should probably contain at least the following descriptions:

- Neuropathic or neuroischemic or ischemic
- Infected or not infected *and*
- Superficial or deep

Summary

Describing a wound in the foot of the diabetic patient as a "diabetic foot ulcer" is too vague. It is not a diagnosis and does not give any information on prognosis

Table 4.1 Three Classification Schemes for Foot Ulcers

Meggitt-Wagner System

Grade	Description
0	Pre-ulcerative/high-risk foot
1	Superficial ulcer
2	Deep to tendon, bone, or joint
3	Deep with abscess/osteomyelitis
4	Forefoot gangrene
5	Whole foot gangrene

University of Texas System

Grade	Description	Stage
0	Pre- or post-ulcerative lesion	A–D
1	Superficial	A–D
2	Penetrates to tendon or capsule	A–D
3	Penetrates to bone	A–D

Stages: A = no infection or ischemia; B = infection; C = ischemia; D = infection and ischemia.

PEDIS System

Perfusion	Normal signs/moderate ischemia/critical limb ischemia
Extent	Area in cm^2
Depth	Superficial/subcutaneous, no bone/deep, extends to bone
Infection	No infection/superficial and localized/extensive or deep/systemic involvement
Sensation	Normal/abnormal

and will not guide therapy. Instead, all foot ulcers in diabetic patients should be evaluated after a rigid and standard protocol. Ulcers can be described as follows:

- Neuropathic, neuroischemic, or ischemic, with or without critical limb ischemia
- Superficial or deep
- Infected or not infected

In addition, the following aspects should be summarized:

- Site of the ulcer (e.g., under the head of metatarsal phalangeal joint 1 [MTP1] or on the dorsal side of the toe)
- Extent (preferably in cm^2)
- Immediate cause (e.g., increased biomechanical stress because of prominent MTP1 or an acute trauma from walking barefoot)

These data will provide the basis for the initial diagnosis and are the cornerstones for formulating a management plan.

References

1. Bakker K, Apelqvist J, Schaper NC; International Working Group on Diabetic Foot Editorial Board. Practical guidelines on the management and prevention of the diabetic foot 2011. *Diabetes Metab Res Rev* 2012;28(Suppl. 1):225–231

2. Norgren L, Hiatt WR, Dormandy JA, et al. Inter-Society Consensus for the Management of Peripheral Arterial Disease (TASCII). *Eur J Vasc Endovasc Surg* 2007;33(Suppl. 1):S1–S75

3. Schaper NC, Andros G, Apelqvist J, et al. Diagnosis and treatment of peripheral arterial disease in diabetic patients with a foot ulcer. A progress report of the International Working Group on the Diabetic Foot. *Diabetes Metab Res Rev* 2012;28(Suppl. 1):218–224

4. Lipsky BA, Berendt AR, Cornia PB, et al. Infectious Diseases Society of America clinical practice guideline for the diagnosis and treatment of diabetic foot infections. *Clin Infect Dis* 2012;54:e132–e173

5. Wagner FW. The dysvascular foot: a system for diagnosis and treatment. *Foot Ankle* 1981;2:64–122

6. Armstrong DG, Lavery LA, Harkless LB. Validation of a diabetic wound classification system: the contribution of depth, infection, and ischemia to risk of amputation. *Diabetes Care* 1998;21:855–859

7. Macfarlane RM, Jeffcoate WJ. Classification of diabetic foot ulcers: the S(AD) SAD system. *Diabetic Foot* 1999;2:123–131

8. Schaper NC. Diabetic foot ulcer classification system for research purposes: a progress report on criteria for including patients in research studies. *Diabetes Metab Res Rev* 2004;20(Suppl. 1):S90–S95

5
Offloading the Diabetic Foot Wound

Stephanie C. Wu, DPM, MSc,[1] and David G. Armstrong, DPM, MD, PhD[2]
[1]Rosalind Franklin University of Medicine, North Chicago, IL; and
[2]University of Arizona College of Medicine, Tucson, AZ

The etiology of ulcerations in individuals with diabetes is generally associated with the presence of peripheral neuropathy and cycles of repetitive stress generated during ambulation, which can expose the foot to moderate or high pressure and shear forces.[1] Foot deformities, limited joint mobility, partial foot amputations, and other structural deformities often predispose diabetic patients with peripheral neuropathy to abnormal weight bearing, areas of concentrated pressure, and abnormal shear forces that significantly increase their risk of ulceration.[2-6] Brand[7] theorized that a local inflammatory response, focal tissue ischemia, tissue destruction, and ulceration could occur when these types of forces were applied to a specific area over an extended period of time.[1] Further, the loss of protective sensation voids the ability to adequately respond to a noxious stimulus. This occurrence may lead to a break in the skin analogous to the way one would wear a hole in a stocking. Because there are no current treatments available to completely ameliorate the effects of neuropathy, the present central tenet in both the treatment and prevention of plantar diabetic foot ulcers centers on the redistribution of pressure.[5,8]

Pressure dispersion, commonly referred to as "offloading," is most successful when the pressure forces are spread over a wide area.[9] There is a plethora of offloading modalities available, and "offloading" is probably the most widely reported treatment for plantar diabetic foot ulcers.[10,11] Current literature contains numerous cohort studies and randomized controlled trials that describe healing with offloading (Table 5.1). The purpose of this chapter is to describe the more commonly used offloading modalities and the evidence that supports their use.

Total Contact Casts

Of the myriad of offloading devices, many consider total contact casting to be the gold standard to heal plantar diabetic foot ulcers.[13–15] Plaster casting to treat neuropathic foot wounds was first described by Milroy Paul and later popularized in the United States by Dr. Paul Brand at the Hansen's Disease Center in Carville, Louisiana.[16] The technique has come to be known as total contact casting because it uses a well-molded, minimally padded cast that maintains contact with the entire plantar aspect of the foot and the lower leg. The intimate fit of the cast material to the plantar surface of the foot increases the plantar weight-bearing surface area to help distribute the plantar pressure from one or two distinct areas to the plantar foot as a whole. Total contact casting is quite effective in treating the majority of non-infected, nonischemic plantar diabetic foot wounds, with healing rates ranging from 72 to 100% over a course of 5–7 weeks.[17–25]

Throughout the gait cycle, the average peak plantar pressures are highest in the forefoot, while they generally tend to be less significant in the rearfoot and medial arch. Shaw et al.[26] and our own group[17] have postulated that a large proportion of the pressure reduction realized in the forefoot of the total contact cast (TCC) is transmitted along the cast wall or to the rearfoot. This finding supports the postulate of several authors who have suggested that the TCC is effective because it permits walking by uniformly distributing pressures over the entire plantar surface of the foot.[16–20,27–29] TCCs have been shown to reduce pressure at the site of ulceration by 84–92%.[2] Histologic information also suggests that pressure relief obtained by casting may reduce localized inflammation and enhance reparative processes.[30] TCCs may also help reduce or control edema that can impede healing and potentially protect the foot from infection.[31] However, the most important attribute of the TCC may be its ability to ensure appropriate patient compliance.[11,32] In other words, the device is not easily removable. Therefore, the patient has no option other than to adhere to the regimen prescribed by the clinician.

Table 5.1 Healing Times in Common Offloading Modalities

Offloading Modality	Mean Healing Time	Type of Study	Percent Healed	Type of Wound	Reference
TCC	Forefoot ulcers: 30 days Rearfoot-midfoot ulcers: 63 days	Retrospective cohort	90%	Wagner 1, 2	Myerson et al.[21]
TCC	Forefoot ulcers: 31 days Rearfoot-midfoot ulcers: 42 days	Retrospective cohort	Not reported	Wagner 1, 2, 3	Walker et al.[19]
TCC	40 days	Retrospective cohort	94%	Wagner 1, 2	Birke et al.[51]
TCC	38 days	Retrospective cohort	73%	Wagner 1, 2, 3	Helm et al.[22]
TCC	44 days	Retrospective cohort	82%	Wagner 1, 2	Sinacore et al.[20]
TCC	Midfoot ulcers: 28 days	Retrospective cohort	100%	Wagner 1, 2	Lavery et al.[29]
TCC RCW Half-shoe	34 days 50 days 61 days	RCT	90% 65% 58%	UT 1A	Armstrong et al.[35]
TCC Shoe insole	85 days 65 days	RCT	90% 32%	Wagner 1, 2	Mueller et al.[31]

Table 5.1 Healing Times in Common Offloading Modalities (continued)

Offloading Modality	Mean Healing Time	Type of Study	Percent Healed	Type of Wound	Reference
Removable cast boot	48 days	RCT	35%	UT 1A	Peters et al.[52]
Fiberglass cast shoe	34 days	Retrospective cohort	91%	Wagner 1	Hissink et al.[44]
Fiberglass cast shoe	Not reported	RCT	50% 21%	Wagner 1	Caravaggi et al.[53]
Scotch cast boot	112 days 181 days	Retrospective cohort	80%	Wagner 1, 2, 3	Knowles et al.[54]
Windowed fiberglass cast Half-shoe	69 days 134 days	Prospective cohort	81% 70%	UT 2A UT1A	Ha Van et al.[50]
Custom splint	300 days	Retrospective cohort	Not reported	Not stated	Boninger et al.[55]
Felted foam dressing Half-shoe	75 days 85 days	RCT	Not reported	Wagner 1, 2	Zimny et al.[56]
TCC Padded dressing Healing shoe Walking splint	48 days 36 days 42 days 51 days	Prospective cohort	92% 93% 81% 83%	Wagner 1, 2, 3	Birke et al.[57]
Removable cast boot/ non-removable	42 days 58 days	RCT	83% 52%	UT 1A-2A	Lavery et al.[41]

Offloading Modality	Mean Healing Time	Type of Study	Percent Healed	Type of Wound	Reference
TCC Non-removable boot	35 days 28 days (median)	RCT	74% 80%	UT 1A-2A	Katz et al.[38]
TCC Non-removable boot	46 days 47 days (median)	Prospective cohort	95% 85%	UT 1A-2A	Piaggesi et al.[39]
TCC Pneumatic RCW	48 days 71 days	RCT	83% 79%	Not stated	Caravaggi et al.[58]
TCC Custom temporary footwear	52 days 90 days	RCT	33% 30%	Wagner 1, 2	Van De Weg et al.[59]
TCC RCW	35 days 40 days	RCT	74% 73%	UT1A	Faglia et al.[24]
TCC RCW	95 days 94 days (median)	RCT	82% 42%	Wagner 1, 2	Gutekunst et al.[60]
Healing sandals TCC Shear Walker	62 days 38 days 47 days (median)	RCT	50% 89% 40%	UT 1A-2A	Lavery et al.[25]

RCT, randomized clinical trial. Reprinted with permission from Baronaski and Ayello.[12]

Certainly, the above-described advantages make the TCC an attractive choice to offload the diabetic foot ulcer. However, there are a number of potential negative attributes that may dissuade some clinicians from using this modality. Data from a diabetic foot ulcer management survey and U.S. Wound Registry noted that TCCs were used about 2% of the time across the United States.[15,33] One of the reasons for the underuse of this device may be that the application of TCCs is time-consuming and often requires a learning curve.[15] Most centers do not have a physician or cast technician available with adequate training or experience to apply a TCC safely. Because improper cast application can cause skin irritation and in some cases even frank ulceration, this can be its single biggest negative feature. In addition, TCCs do not allow patients, family members, or health care providers to assess the foot or wound on a daily basis, and TCCs are contraindicated in cases of soft tissue infections or osteomyelitis. Other patient complaints may include difficulty sleeping comfortably as well as bathing difficulties when avoiding getting the cast wet. TCCs may also exacerbate postural instability.[34]

Removable Cast Walkers

Removable cast walkers (RCWs) offer several advantages over the traditional TCC. Removable walkers are, as their name implies, easily removed for self-inspection of the wound and application of topical therapies that require frequent administration. The cost of a cast technician's time to apply a new cast and the cost of materials are also significantly reduced when the offloading device can be easily reused.[24] Patients can bathe and sleep more comfortably. Because they are removable, RCWs can be used for infected wounds as well as superficial ulcers.

Although data from gait lab studies suggest that pressure reduction for certain RCWs is equivalent to that of TCCs, results of randomized clinical studies do not show equivalent clinical outcomes. A meta-analysis of the studies that compared the use of non-removable devices with the RCW showed a trend favoring the non-removable devices.[11] In a study that compared the efficacy of TCCs, RCWs, and half-shoes to heal diabetic foot ulcerations, a significantly higher proportion of patients healed by 12 weeks in the TCC group than with the two other modalities, removable cast boots and half-shoes.[35]

The reason people do not heal as well in removable devices is that they are removable. The best feature of the RCW is also, paradoxically, its potential downfall. The ability to remove the device eliminates the element of "forced compliance," which is the finest attribute of the TCC. Patients may remove the RCW for dressing changes, sleeping, and showers, but they may also choose to use the walker only when they leave the house or walk long distances. Armstrong et al.[36] found that the RCW was used for only 28% of a patient's total daily activity. In individuals who have lost the gift of pain secondary to neuropathy, patients will generally do what feels best.[36] A heavy boot may not feel comfortable to many patients, leading ultimately to noncompliance.

Instant Total Contact Cast

It would be ideal to be able to take the clinical efficacy of the TCC and combine it with the relative ease of application of the RCW.[23] Armstrong et al.[37] have termed an innovative approach to use the RCW with enhanced compliance: the instant total contact cast (iTCC). The iTCC involves simply wrapping a RCW with a single layer of cohesive bandage, elastoplast, or casting tape. An iTCC may best address the limitations of both a traditional TCC and RCW, in that it may enforce compliance and pressure redistribution while allowing for ease of application and examination of the ulcer when needed. Two additional studies were subsequently conducted to test the wound-healing efficacy of the iTCC. The first randomized controlled study compared the standard TCC with an iTCC.[38] The study found no differences in healing rates and the mean healing time between patients who received the TCC versus the iTCC. There were also no differences in complications between the two groups. However, the cost in materials and personnel was much lower for the iTCC than the TCC. The study concluded that the iTCC is not only equally efficacious in healing diabetic foot ulcers, when compared with the TCC, but is quicker, easier, and more cost-effective than the TCC.[38]

A parallel study[14] that compared the effectiveness of an RCW and an iTCC in the healing of neuropathic diabetic foot ulcerations showed comparable results. The study found that a significantly higher proportion of patients healed in the iTCC group when compared with the RCW group. Of the patients who healed, individuals treated with the iTCC healed significantly faster.[14] A prospective randomized trial found equivalent healing efficacy between the iTCC and TCC, while favoring the iTCC in terms of cost reduction, practicability, patient satisfaction, and time required for application.[39] Data from a recent meta-analysis showed TCCs and iTCCs to be equally effective at achieving complete healing of diabetic foot ulcers.[11] Interestingly, patients using a non-removable device were found to take 22% fewer steps than those using a RCW and 59% fewer steps than patients using a therapeutic shoe.[35] This reduced activity can further help increase the pressure mitigation effect of the non-removable devices and increase their effectiveness in diabetic ulcer healing.

Half-Shoes (Forefoot Offloading Shoes)

Originally designed to decrease pressure on the forefoot postoperatively,[40] the half-shoe has become quite popular for treating diabetic foot wounds. These devices are inexpensive and easy to apply. Chantelau and coworkers retrospectively evaluated 22 patients treated with half-shoes, compared with 26 patients who received "routine wound care" and crutch-assisted gait. The results indicated that the median time to healing was faster with the half-shoe (70 vs. 118 days) and that patients developed fewer serious infections requiring hospitalization (4 vs. 41%).[40] In a gait lab study comparing half-shoes to TCCs and RCWs, half-shoes were much less effective at reducing pressure than TCCs and RCWs.[41] This is echoed in the results of a randomized controlled trial that found the healing efficacy of TCCs, RCWs, and half-shoes to be 89.5, 65.0, and 58.3%, respectively.[35] A recent systematic review assessing the effectiveness of footwear and other removable offloading devices in the treatment of diabetic foot ulcers found half-shoes to be the second least effective intervention.[42]

Just as is the case with RCWs and the other modalities described in this review, studies evaluating outcomes, patient satisfaction, costs, and complications are needed to study this modality completely, compared with other frequently used devices.

Healing Sandals

Several authors have advocated the use of various forms of "healing sandals" to treat diabetic foot ulcers. Application of a rigid rocker to the sole of a specially designed sandal may limit dorsiflexion of the metatarsophalangeal joints, thereby reducing the pressure and pressure-time integral at the site of ulceration. In addition, the molded nature of a "healing sandal" provides a greater distribution of metatarsal head pressures. Healing sandals are lightweight, stable, and reusable. However, they require a significant amount of time and experience to produce the rigid sole rocker design and other modifications. Most facilities will not have the time or expertise to modify these devices. Finally, these devices do not work as well as many other modalities that take less effort to produce.[43] The results of a recent randomized controlled trial found the healing efficacy of healing sandals to be 50%, statistically lower than the healing efficacy of 89% seen with TCC.[25]

In the late 1990s, a cross between a healing sandal and an RCW was introduced. This device, known as the MABAL shoe, is removable, but perhaps maintains more contact with the foot than a standard healing sandal. In a study by Hissink et al.,[44] the MABAL shoe showed a similar time to healing when compared with studies of total contact casting. However, the MABAL shoe also has many of the downfalls of the contact cast and healing sandal, since it requires special expertise for its fabrication and application.

Shoe Modifications

"Felted foam," fashioned by fixing a bi-layered felt-foam pad over the plantar aspect of the foot with an aperture corresponding to the site of ulceration, and shoe modifications are frequently used to offload the foot. There are only anecdotal reports of success using this approach.[45] Gait lab studies suggest that these felt and foam accommodative dressings are not as effective as RCWs or TCCs to reduce peak foot pressures in patients with diabetic foot ulcers.[46] Fleischli and colleagues conducted a gait lab study comparing the offloading ability of TCC, half-shoe, RCW, rigid postoperative shoe, and felted foam accommodative dressing. The results of this project suggested that TCCs and certain RCWs achieved the best reduction of plantar pressures at the site of neuropathic ulcerations. The half-shoe finished a distant third, followed by the felted foam dressings and surgical shoes. However, when compared to the half-shoe, Zimny and colleagues found statistically significant difference in time to healing favoring the felted foam dressing.[47] Although less effective than the TCC, felted foam may have some benefits in that it can be applied in the presence of mild to moderate infection, allows for frequent dressing changes, and can be applied rapidly.[48] Of note is that the felted foam dressing may need to be replaced every 3 days, since a previous study showed that the felted foam was effective at reducing the peak plantar pressure at the ulcerations site by about 70% for the initial 3 days, but lost its ability to mitigate pressure on day 4.[49]

There are real concerns that an aperture applied around the wound based solely on visual cues (without gait laboratory confirmation) may increase shear and vertical forces at the wound's periphery secondary to the "edge effect."[17]

Felted foam and shoe modifications may be popular because patients are resistant to casts or the extra costs associated with RCWs. Clinicians are therefore compelled to use alternative pressure mitigation methods such as shoe modifications. Shoe modifications are often less costly than other modalities and are reimbursable. Further, patients are often more tolerant of the slight modifications made to shoes with which they are most familiar.

Crutches, Walkers, and Wheelchairs

It would stand to reason that completely offloading a foot with crutches, walkers, or wheelchairs would be effective in promoting healing in the diabetic wound. However, the vast majority of patients for whom these devices are prescribed do not have the upper-body strength, endurance, or willpower to use these devices.[38] Additionally, some of these devices can place the contralateral limb at risk for ulceration by increasing pressure to the unaffected side.[41] Most patients' domiciles are not designed for wheelchair access, thus reducing their utility in the place where they may be most active—at home.

Therapeutic Footwear (Depth Inlay Shoes)

Many patients are prescribed therapeutic shoes in an effort to assist in pressure reduction and wound healing. However, therapeutic shoes have not proven to be effective in this role. A recent systematic review found currently available therapeutic shoes to be the least effective intervention followed by half or heel relief shoes.[42] Gait lab studies suggest that therapeutic shoes allow much greater pressure in areas of the forefoot, compared with TCCs and some RCWs.[2] In a clinical controlled trial where a therapeutic shoe and insole were used as the control group, only about 31% of patients healed, compared with the TCC, where about 90% of the ulcers healed.[31] Moreover, therapeutic shoes can be easily removed, thereby further reducing the healing efficacy due to patient noncompliance.[11] Ha Van et al.[50] found that less than half of the patients complied with the use of therapeutic shoes versus almost total enforced compliance with the TCC. We may therefore postulate that the true value of therapeutic shoes and insoles is in the prevention of ulceration, not during active ulceration. Therapeutic shoes and insoles are much less effective than other methods to offload the foot. These devices may be preferred in patients with poor postural stability, since these patients are unable to walk safely in a device that restricts their balance.

In conclusion, the results of several recent meta-analyses demonstrate that non-removable offloading devices, regardless of the type, prove to be the most effective pressure mitigation interventions for healing diabetic foot ulcers.[11,42,48] However, the criteria for selection of an offloading device includes efficacy, safety, availability, cost, and patient acceptance and compliance. The recent history of the treatment of wounds in general—and of diabetic wounds specifically—has been marked by some exciting advances on the high-tech front; it is in fact the low-tech systematic aspects of care that must assume priority. We have often been heard saying, "It's not what one puts on a wound that heals it, but what one takes off." To diminish the detrimental consequences associated with diabetic foot ulcers, a consistent standard of care must be provided. Appropriate wound care, debridement, and patient compliance to pressure reduction are the cornerstones of treatment.

References

1. Brand PW. The insensitive foot (including leprosy). In *Disorders of the Foot and Ankle*. 2nd ed. Jahss M, Ed. Philadelphia, Saunders, 1991, p. 2170–2175

2. Lavery LA, Vela SA, Lavery DC, Quebedeaux TL. Reducing dynamic foot pressures in high-risk diabetic subjects with foot ulcerations: a comparison of treatments. *Diabetes Care* 1996;19:818–821

3. Lavery LA, Lavery DC, Quebedeax-Farnham TL. Increased foot pressures after great toe amputation in diabetes. *Diabetes Care* 1995; 18:1460–1462

4. Knowles A, Armstrong DG, Hayat SA, et al. Offloading diabetic foot wound using the scotchcast boot: a retrospective study. *Ostomy Wound Manage* 2002:48;50–53

5. Bell D. Evidence-based rationale for offloading treatment modalities. *Surg Technol Int* 2008;17:113–117

6. Waaijman R, de Haart M, Arts ML, et al. Risk factors for plantar foot ulcer recurrence in neuropathic diabetic patients. *Diabetes Care* 2014; 37:1697–1705

7. Brand PW. The diabetic foot. In *Diabetes Mellitus, Theory and Practice*. 3rd ed. Ellenberg M, Rifkin H, Eds. New York, Medical Examination Publishing, 1983, p. 803–828

8. Bus SA. Priorities in offloading the diabetic foot. *Diabetes Metab Res Rev.* 2012;28(Suppl. 1):54–59

9. Cavanagh PR, Bus SA. Off-loading the diabetic foot for ulcer prevention and healing. *J Vasc Surg* 2010;52:37S–43S

10. Bus SA, Valk GD, van Deursen RW, et al. The effectiveness of footwear and offloading interventions to prevent and heal foot ulcers and reduce plantar pressure in diabetes: a systematic review. *Diabetes Metab Res Rev* 2008;24(Suppl. 1):S162–S180

11. Morona JK, Buckley ES, Jones S, et al. Comparison of the clinical effectiveness of different off-loading devices for the treatment of neuropathic foot ulcers in patients with diabetes: a systematic review and meta-analysis. *Diabetes Metab Res Rev* 2013;29:183–193

12. Baronaski S, Ayello EA. *Wound Care Essentials: Practice Principles*. 2nd ed. Baltimore, MD, Lippincott Williams & Wilkins, 2007

13. Apelqvist J, Bakker K, van Houtum WH, et al. International consensus and practical guidelines on the management and the prevention of the diabetic foot: International Working Group on the Diabetic Foot. *Diabetes Metab Res Rev* 2000;6(Suppl. 1):S84–S92

14. Armstrong DG, Lavery LA, Wu S, Boulton AJ. Evaluation of removable and irremovable cast walkers in the healing of diabetic foot wounds: a randomized controlled trial. *Diabetes Care* 2005;28:551–554

15. Wu SC, Jensen JL, Weber AK, et al. Use of pressure offloading devices in diabetic foot ulcers: do we practice what we preach? *Diabetes Care* 2008;31:2118–2119

16. Coleman W, Brand PW, Birke JA. The total contact cast, a therapy for plantar ulceration on insensitive feet. *J Am Podiatr Med Assoc* 1984;74:548–552

17. Armstrong DG, Athanasiou KA. The edge effect: how and why wounds grow in size and depth. *Clin Podiatr Med Surg* 1998;15:105–108

18. Walker SC, Helm PA, Pulliam G. Chronic diabetic neuropathic foot ulcerations and total contact casting: healing effectiveness and outcome probability (Abstract). *Arch Phys Med Rehabil* 1985;66:574

19. Walker SC, Helm PA, Pulliam G. Total contact casting and chronic diabetic neuropathic foot ulcerations: healing rates by wound location. *Arch Phys Med Rehabil* 1987;68:217–221

20. Sinacore DR, Mueller MJ, Diamond JE. Diabetic plantar ulcers treated by total contact casting. *Phys Ther* 1987;67:1543–1547

21. Myerson M, Papa J, Eaton K, Wilson K. The total contact cast for management of neuropathic plantar ulceration of the foot. *J Bone Joint Surg Am* 1992;74A:261–269

22. Helm PA, Walker SC, Pulliam G. Total contact casting in diabetic patients with neuropathic foot ulcerations. *Arch Phys Med Rehabil* 1984;65:691–693

23. Ganguly S, Chakraborty K, Mandal PK, et al. A comparative study between total contact casting and conventional dressings in the non-surgical management of diabetic plantar foot ulcers. *J Indian Med Assoc* 2008;106:237–239, 244

24. Faglia E, Caravaggi C, Clerici G, et al. Effectiveness of removable walker cast versus nonremovable fiberglass off-bearing cast in the healing of diabetic plantar foot ulcer: a randomized controlled trial. *Diabetes Care* 2010;33:1419–1423

25. Lavery LA, Higgins KR, La Fontaine J, et al. Randomised clinical trial to compare total contact casts, healing sandals and a shear-reducing removable boot to heal diabetic foot ulcers. *Int Wound J* doi: 10.1111/iwj.12213. Epub 21 Feb 2014

26. Shaw JE, Hsi WL, Ulbrecht JS, et al. The mechanism of plantar unloading in total contact casts: implications for design and clinical use. *Foot Ankle Int* 1997;18:809–817

27. Boulton AJM, Bowker JH, Gadia M, et al. Use of plaster casts in the management of diabetic neuropathic foot ulcers. *Diabetes Care* 1986;9:149–152

28. Kominsky SJ. The ambulatory total contact cast. In *The High Risk Foot in Diabetes Mellitus.* 1st ed. Frykberg RG, Ed. New York, Churchill Livingstone, 1991, p. 449–455

29. Lavery LA, Armstrong DG, Walker SC. Healing rates of diabetic foot ulcers associated with midfoot fracture due to Charcot's arthropathy. *Diabet Med* 1997;14:46–49

30. Piaggesi A, Viacava P, Rizzo L, et al. Semiquantitative analysis of the histopathological features of the neuropathic foot ulcer: effects of pressure relief. *Diabetes Care* 2003;26:3123–3128

31. Mueller MJ, Diamond JE, Sinacore DR, et al. Total contact casting in treatment of diabetic plantar ulcers: controlled clinical trial. *Diabetes Care* 1989;12:384–388

32. Wu SC, Driver VR, Wrobel JS, Armstrong DG. Foot ulcers in the diabetic patient, prevention and treatment. *Vasc Health Risk Manag* 2007;3:65–76

33. Fife CE, Carter MJ, Walker D, et al. Diabetic foot ulcer off-loading: the gap between evidence and practice: data from the US Wound Registry. *Adv Skin Wound Care* 2014;27:310–316

34. Lavery LA, Fleishli JG, Laughlin TJ, et al. Is postural instability exacerbated by off-loading devices in high risk diabetics with foot ulcers? *Ostomy Wound Manage* 1998;44:26–32, 34

35. Armstrong DG, Nguyen HC, Lavery LA, et al. Off-loading the diabetic foot wound: a randomized clinical trial. *Diabetes Care* 2001;24:1019–1022

36. Armstrong DG, Lavery LA, Kimbriel HR, et al. Activity patterns of patients with diabetic foot ulceration: patients with active ulceration may not adhere to a standard pressure off-loading regimen. *Diabetes Care* 2003;26:2595–2597

37. Armstrong DG, Short B, Espensen EH, et al. Technique for fabrication of an "instant total-contact cast" for treatment of neuropathic diabetic foot ulcers. *J Am Podiatr Med Assoc* 2002;92:405–408

38. Katz IA, Harlan A, Miranda-Palma B, et al. A randomized trial of two irremovable off-loading devices in the management of plantar neuropathic diabetic foot ulcers. *Diabetes Care* 2005;28:555–559

39. Piaggesi A, Macchiarini S, Rizzo L, et al. An off-the-shelf instant contact casting device for the management of diabetic foot ulcers: a randomized prospective trial versus traditional fiberglass cast. *Diabetes Care* 2007;30:586–590

40. Chantelau E, Breuer U, Leisch AC, et al. Outpatient treatment of unilateral diabetic foot ulcers with 'half shoes.' *Diabet Med* 1993;10:267–270

41. Lavery LA, Vela SA, Lavery DC, Quebedeaux TL. Reducing dynamic foot pressures in high-risk diabetic subjects with foot ulcerations: a comparison of treatments. *Diabetes Care* 1996;19:818–821

42. Healy A, Naemi R, Chockalingam N. The effectiveness of footwear and other removable off-loading devices in the treatment of diabetic foot ulcers: a systematic review. *Curr Diabetes Rev* 2014;10:215–230

43. Giacalone VF, Armstrong DG, Ashry HR, et al. A quantitative assessment of healing sandals and postoperative shoes in offloading diabetic foot. *J Foot Ankle Surg* 1997;36:28–30

44. Hissink RJ, Manning HA, van Baal JG. The MABAL shoe, an alternative method in contact casting for the treatment of neuropathic diabetic foot ulcers. *Foot Ankle Int* 2000;21:320–323

45. Guzman B, Fisher G, Palladino SJ, Stavosky JW. Pressure-removing strategies in neuropathic ulcer therapy. *Clin Pod Med Surg* 1994;11:339–353

46. Fleischli JG, Lavery LA, Vela SA, et al. 1997 William J. Stickel Bronze Award: Comparison of strategies for reducing pressure at the site of neuropathic ulcers. *J Am Podiatr Med Assoc* 1997;87:466–472

47. Zimny S, Schatz H, Pfohl U. The effects of applied felted foam on wound healing and healing times in the therapy of neuropathic diabetic foot ulcers. *Diabet Med* 2003;20:622–625

48. Lewis J, Lipp A. Pressure-relieving interventions for treatment diabetic foot ulcers. *Cochrane Database Syst Rev.* 1:CD002302. doi:10.1002/14651858.CD002302.pub2. Epub 31 Jan 2013

49. Zimny S, Reinsch B, Schatz H, Pfohl M. Effects of felted foam on plantar pressures in the treatment of neuropathic diabetic foot ulcers. *Diabetes Care* 2001;24:2153–2154

50. Ha Van G, Siney H, Hartmann-Heurtier A, et al. Nonremovable, windowed, fiberglass cast boot in the treatment of diabetic plantar ulcers: efficacy, safety, and compliance. *Diabetes Care* 2003;26:2848–2852

51. Birke JA, Novick A, Patout CA, Coleman WC. Healing rates of plantar ulcers in leprosy and diabetes. *Lepr Rev* 1992;63:365–374

52. Peters EJ, Lavery LA, Armstrong DG, Fleischli JG. Electric stimulation as an adjunct to heal diabetic foot ulcers: a randomized clinical trial. *Arch Phys Med Rehabil* 2001;82:721–725

53. Caravaggi C, Faglia E, De Giglio R, et al. Effectiveness and safety of a nonremovable fiberglass off-bearing cast versus a therapeutic shoe in the treatment of neuropathic foot ulcers: a randomized study. *Diabetes Care* 2000;23:1746–1751

54. Knowles EA, Armstrong DG, Hayat SA, et al. Offloading diabetic foot wounds using the scotchcast boot: a retrospective study. *Ostomy Wound Manage* 2002;48:50–53

55. Boninger ML, Leonard JA Jr. Use of bivalved ankle-foot orthosis in neuropathic foot and ankle lesions. *J Rehabil Res Dev* 1996;33:16–22

56. Zimny S, Meyer MF, Schatz H, Pfohl M. Applied felted foam for plantar pressure relief is an efficient therapy in neuropathic diabetic foot ulcers. *Exp Clin Endocrinol Diabetes* 2002;110:325–328

57. Birke JA, Pavich MA, Patout CA, Horswell R. Comparison of forefoot ulcer healing using alternative off-loading methods in patients with diabetes mellitus. *Adv Skin Wound Care* 2002;15:210–215

58. Caravaggi C, Sganzaroli A, Fabbi M, et al. Nonwindowed nonremovable fiberglass off-loading cast versus removable pneumatic cast (AircastXP Diabetic Walker) in the treatment of neuropathic noninfected plantar ulcers. *Diabetes Care* 2007;30:2577–2578

59. Van De Weg FB, Van Der Windt DA, Vahl AC. Wound healing: total contact cast vs. custom made temporary foot-wear for patients with diabetic foot ulceration. *Prosthet Orthot Int* 2008;32:3–11

60. Gutekunst DJ, Hastings MK, Bohnert KL, et al. Removable cast walker boots yield greater forefoot off-loading than total contact casts. *Clinical Biomechanics* 2011;26:649–654

Suggested Readings

Armstrong DG, Lavery LA, Bushman TR. Peak foot pressures influence healing time of diabetic ulcers treated with total contact casting. *J Rehabil Res Dev* 1998;35:1–5

6
Debridement of the Diabetic Foot

Andrew J. Meyr, DPM[1]; John S. Steinberg, DPM[2]; Paul Kim, DPM[2]; and
Christopher E. Attinger, MD[2]
[1]*Department of Podiatric Surgery, Temple University of Podiatric Medicine,
Philadelphia, PA; and [2]Department of Surgery, Division of Plastic Surgery,
Georgetown University of Medicine, Washington, DC*

Acute wounds should proceed quickly and uneventfully through the normal stages of the body's natural healing process: inflammation, proliferation, and maturation.[1] This process is usually a linear pathway, with a distinct start point (wound formation) and a clear endpoint (wound closure). Unfortunately, patients with diabetes are at an increased risk for the development of chronic wounds. This result is largely due to a combination of neuropathy and joint and tendon stiffness that alters the biomechanics sufficiently, causing tissue breakdown to occur. In these situations, the normal physiology of the linear pathway is transformed into the pathophysiology of a chronic cycle, without a clear wound-closure endpoint. A chronic wound is arrested in one of the healing stages (usually the inflammatory stage) and cannot progress further. Diabetic wounds that do not progress toward closure at a consistent rate—a reduction in wound volume by an average of ~10–15% per week[2]—should be actively recognized as chronic wounds and treated appropriately.

Although there are many potential reasons for the development of chronic wounds in diabetic patients, the pathophysiological healing processes of the chronic wound should not be overlooked.[3] Necrotic tissue, foreign material, and bacteria in a wound impede the body's attempt to heal by producing or stimulating the production of abnormal metalloproteases such as col-

DOI: 10.2337/9781580405706.06

lagenases and elastases. These metalloproteases then overwhelm the building blocks—chemoattractants, growth factors, and mitogens—needed for normal wound healing. This hostile environment enables bacteria to proliferate. The bacteria further inhibit healing by producing their own destructive enzymes and by consuming the local resources necessary for healing (oxygen, nutrition, and building blocks).

In addition, the wound base and wound edges are specifically affected by this pathophysiology. Bacteria inhibit healing by producing a biofilm for their own protection. This biofilm is an extracellular matrix that irreversibly binds to the wound base, is inflammatory to the surrounding material, and may cause resistance to traditional therapeutic interventions.[4] The biofilm spreads along the vessels feeding the base of the wound and can be as deep as 4 mm below the surface of the wound. In chronic wounds, it is often necessary to physically reduce the amount of biofilm from the wound base to affect healing. In addition, cells at the wound edge develop a tendency to become senescent, or with decreased ability to perform the DNA replication needed for continued healing.[5] Senescent cells at the wound edge may also need to be physically removed to stimulate the acute healing processes.

Removing necrotic tissue, foreign material, and bacteria, as well as the biofilm and senescent cells from a wound, occurs through the process known as "debridement." This initial step is critical in allowing the wound to regain the normal physiology of healing in a timely fashion. Debriding the chronic wound to normal tissue physically converts it into an acute wound that can then progress through the normal phases of healing.[6-8]

The largest impediment to successful debridement is medical personnel's fear of debridement. That is due to two factors: 1) how to close the wound once it has been successfully debrided and 2) the fear of debriding adequately. For that reason, it is recommended that treating the diabetic foot is done by a team that involves a reconstructive surgeon who can close the wound once it has been adequately debrided. Debriding too little does not get rid of the infection and debriding too much may sacrifice critical portions of the foot so that a biomechanically stable foot cannot be reconstructed.

Timing of a Debridement

Ischemia and infection are two factors that may influence the timing of a debridement. When dealing with gangrene in the ischemic limb, the timing between debridement and revascularization is important. When faced with wet gangrene or abscess formation in an ischemic limb, the wound should be debrided immediately, regardless of the need for revascularization. The leg should then be revascularized as soon as possible thereafter. But if there is dry gangrene and no cellulitis, the limb should be revascularized first.

It can take anywhere from a few days up to as many as 4 weeks after revascularization to optimize blood flow to the foot.[9] Part of this variability depends on which type of vascular procedure is performed, whether a bypass (relatively quicker optimization of blood flow) or an endovascular procedure (relatively slower optimization). To avoid debriding potentially viable tissue during this time, debridement should be delayed, if possible, until the wound has developed maximal blood flow from the procedure. However, if the dry gangrene converts to wet gangrene before full tissue revascularization has occurred, the gangrene should be immediately debrided.

If dry gangrene is present in a vascularized limb, closely observe for evidence of new tissue growth underneath the eschar. If there is evidence of new tissue growth, then observe the gangrene until it falls off or converts to wet gangrene. If there is no evidence of new tissue growth or healing, then it should be debrided.

Surgical Debridement

When debriding, use atraumatic surgical techniques to avoid damaging the healthy tissue left behind. Such tissue will be the future source of growth factors, nutrients, and building blocks required for subsequent healing, and it should be protected. To leave a maximal amount of viable tissue behind, avoid traumatizing techniques such as crushing the skin edges with forceps or clamps, burning tissue with electrocautery, or tying off large segments of tissue with sutures.

The principal debriding technique consists of removing the grossly contaminated or ischemic tissue en masse. Use any appropriate surgical instrument, including a surgical blade, Mayo scissors, curettes, and rongeurs. However, as viable tissue is approached, slice thin layer of tissue after thin layer of tissue until only normal tissue remains. This technique minimizes the amount of viable tissue sacrificed while ensuring that the tissue left behind will be healthy. When assessing whether normal tissue has been reached, use the color of the tissue as a guide: normal yellow of fat or bone, white fascia or tendon, and red muscle. Any other color usual means residual dead or abnormal tissue that needs to be further debrided.

The basic tools of debridement used in an office include pickups, blades, scissors, and curettes. Surgical instruments, not disposable suture removal kits, are recommended because the latter are usually dull, and they crush and damage the normal tissue left behind. Grasp the tissue to be removed with the pickup, and use a #10 or #20 blade to slice off tissue, thin layer by thin layer (Fig. 6.1), until healthy tissue is reached. Change surgical blades frequently, as they dull quickly. Curettes with sharp edges are helpful for removing the proteinaceous coagulum that accumulates on top of both fresh and chronic granulation tissue (Fig. 6.2A and B) but are not effective in getting rid of biofilm. A hydrosurgical debrider (discussed below) does shave off tissue much like a planer and reduces biofilm by greater than 2 logs of biofilm. Rongeurs are useful for removing hard-to-reach soft tissue and for debriding bone. A pneumatic or electrical sagittal saw can serially saw off bone until you reach normal cortex and marrow. Cutting burrs and rasps permit fine debridement of the bone surface until the telltale punctate bleeding at the remaining bone surface is seen.

A useful technique to ensure that the entire surface of the wound is identified, including nooks and crannies, is to paint the wound surface with methylene blue dye. Once all the dye has been surgically debrided, it will be clear if the surface biofilm has been debrided. Again, debriding should continue until normal tissue colors are reached. When dealing with the indurated walls of a chronic wound, usually slicing off only 1–2 mm thickness of that wall gets you to soft normal tissue. When preparing a granulating bed for a skin graft, there is usually biofilm that lies at the base of the micro-papilla of the granulation tissue. The granulation tissue has to be debrided to the base of the wound until there is a yellow base. The blood flow that fed the granulation tissue is still there, but the biofilm at the base of the wound is gone. This step ensures a higher skin graft take.

In addition to standard surgical tools, a hydrosurgical debrider that uses a saline jet with up to 15,000 psi to debride tissue is also available. The Venturi effect caused by this high-pressure water jet evacuates the tissue into the stream of saline, thus separating it from underlying tissue. This debrider works rapidly to shave off thin slice after thin slice of tissue with minimal surrounding tissue trauma and can greatly expedite difficult debridement tasks. It does reduce biofilm by greater than 2 logs of biofilm.

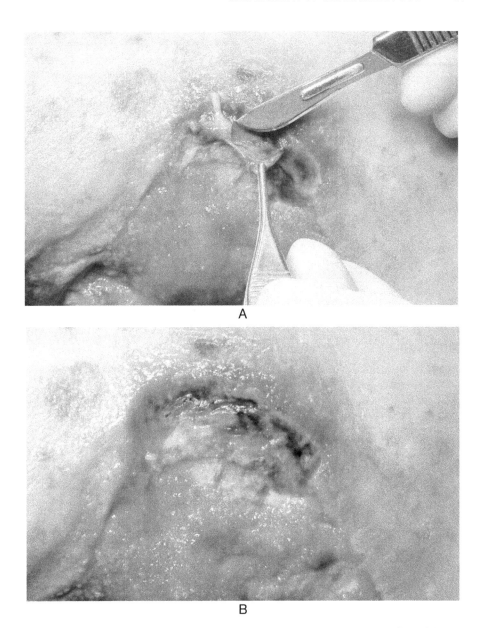

A

B

Figure 6.1—Remove thin slices of necrotic tissue, one layer at a time (A). The appearance of clotted veins in the tissue (B) signifies that further debridement (C—next page) is needed. Continue debriding until only viable tissue remains (D—next page). Note that the skin edges have also been resected. To ensure that the entire surface of the wound has been removed, one might want to paint the surface of the wound first with methylene blue dye and debride until no blue remains.

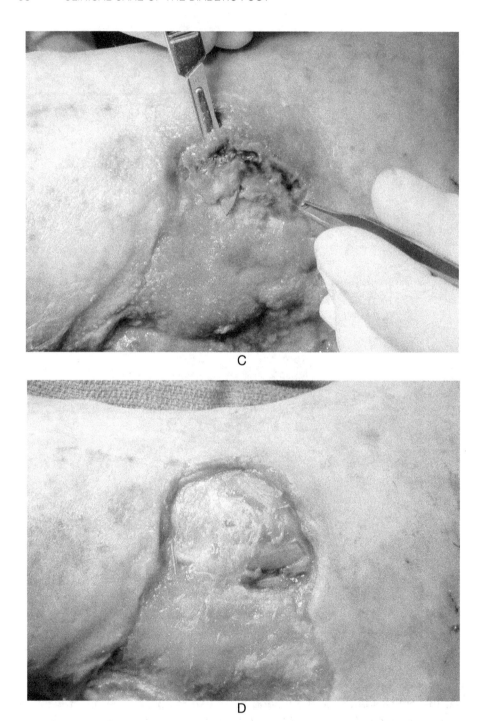

C

D

Figure 6.1—continued

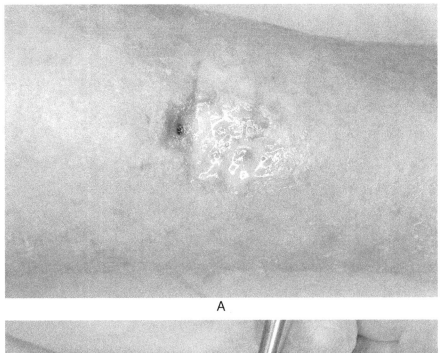

A

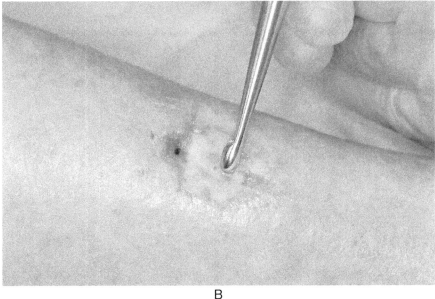

B

Figure 6.2—Any thick coagulum (A) that covers chronic and acute wounds should be curetted off (B—this page—and C—next page) because it contains metalloproteases that inhibit healing. After the wound is adequately curetted, only healthy granulating tissue should remain (D—next page). But curetting only removes 0.5 logs of biofilm and should not be relied on for biofilm removal.

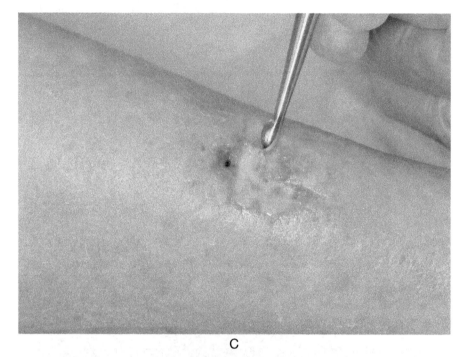

C

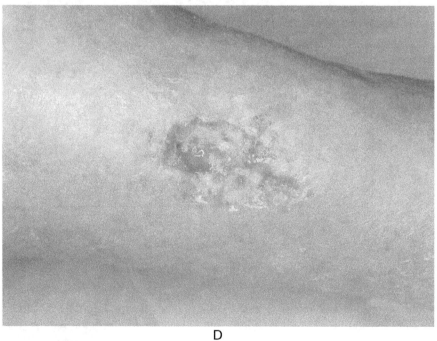

D

Figure 6.2—continued

Additionally, ultrasound-based technologies are also available for debridement of problem wounds. These instruments come in a variety of forms and vary in their aggressiveness for actual tissue removal versus wound bed preparation focus. These technologies have shown promise in optimizing the debridements performed just before application of a split thickness skin graft of bioengineered alternative tissues. They may also be more effective in getting rid of biofilm.

Debriding Skin

Remove nonviable skin as soon as possible. If the border between live and dead tissue is clearly demarcated, excise the skin along that border. If the border is not obvious, start at the center and remove concentric circles of skin until bleeding tissue is reached. When excising skin, look for bleeding at the normal skin edge. Clotted venules at the skin edge indicate that the local microcirculation has been completely interrupted and that further excision is necessary. The cutaneous debridement is adequate when there is normal arterial and venous bleeding at the edge of the wound. In the case of chronic wounds, it is recommended to excise a 2- to 4-mm rim around the periphery of the wound to remove the senescent cells that are impeding healing.

Debriding Subcutaneous Tissue

Subcutaneous tissue consists of fat, superficial nerves, and a relatively decreased concentration of blood vessels compared with the skin. Because of the relative hypovascularity in the subcutaneous fat, bleeding at the tissue's edge is not always a reliable indicator of viability. Healthy fat has a shiny yellow color and is soft and resilient. Dead fat has a gray pallor and is hard and not pliable. Debride this layer until soft, pliable, yellow, and normal-appearing fat is reached. After debridement, keep fat in a moist environment to prevent desiccation.

To minimize damage to the surrounding tissue, coagulate the small blood vessels using bipolar cautery. Ligate vessels if they are larger than 2–3 mm. Ligaclips are the least reactive foreign body material for this purpose. If a suture is used for ligation, a small-diameter monofilament will minimize the risk of further inflammatory response and infection.

Debriding Fascia, Tendon, and Muscle

Healthy fascia has a hard, white, and glistening appearance. When dead, it looks dull, soft, and stringy and may be in the process of liquefying. Debride all necrotic fascia until it is solid, normal-looking, and bleeding. It is important to note that the viable fascia must be kept moist during the post-debridement period to avoid desiccation.

Infected and necrotic tendon looks dull, soft, and partially liquefied. To ensure that any hidden necrotic tendon is also removed, make a proximal and distal incision along the path of the exposed tendon. When the extensor tendons on the dorsum of the foot become exposed, it is hard to preserve them unless they are quickly covered with healthy tissue. If these tendons remain in place while the wound progresses and is ready to be closed, they usually become infected and will impede further healing until they are removed. With the larger Achilles or anterior tibial tendon, debride only the portion that is necrotic or infected. Leave any hard and shiny tendon intact. The remaining tendon must be kept moist and clean throughout the granulation process until a skin graft can be applied. Granulation formulation can be accelerated with the use of negative pressure wound therapy (first cover the tendon with a Vaseline mesh gauze or silicone sheeting), a dermal template, bioengineered alternative tissues, or the combined use of topical growth factor and hyperbaric oxygen.

Examine the underlying muscle. Healthy muscle has a bright red, shiny, and resilient appearance, and it contracts when grasped with forceps or touched with cautery. The muscle in neuropathic patients may have a pale, possibly yellowish color, and may appear nonviable. However, it will have some tone, and it will bleed when cut. Frankly dead muscle will be swollen, dull, and grainy when palpated, and it falls apart when pinched. If the viability of the muscle is questionable, err on the side of caution, and remove only what is not bleeding and appears dead.

Debriding Bone

The key to the debridement of bone is to remove only what is dead and infected and to leave behind any bone that is hard and bleeding. Be careful not to shatter proximal viable bone. With this in mind, power tools are safer to use than rongeurs or chisels. The best way to debride the osteomyelitic smaller long bones (phalanges or metatarsals) is to cut small slices serially with a sagittal saw until healthy bone is reached. In the larger bones, use a cutting burr to remove thin layer by thin layer of bone until punctate bleeding (paprika sign) is seen. Copiously irrigate to ensure that the heat generated by the burr does not damage the healthy bone. Continue debriding until you reach marrow that is bleeding and appears normal.

Obtain clean cultures of normal bone left behind after debridement, as well as those of the debrided osteomyelitic bone. Once all infected bone is removed and only bleeding, healthy bone remains, and assuming that the surrounding soft tissue is also healthy, the wound is ready to close. The culture results of the clean bone after debridement help determine the length of antibiotic therapy. A longer course of antibiotics (6–8 weeks) is required if you suspect that the bone left behind still harbors osteomyelitis.[10] However, a greatly shortened course of antibiotics (1 week) is necessary after wound closure when only healthy, non-infected bone is left behind.

Nonsurgical Modes of Debridement

Certainly not all patients are surgical candidates, and there are several nonsurgical modes of debridement available for these patients. Wet-to-dry dressings, where the saline-moistened gauze is allowed to dry on the wound and then is physically peeled off, are a standard mechanical debriding dressing. Although this effectively removes dead tissue, it can lead to wound desiccation, can harm the viable tissue left behind, and is painful in the sensate patient. There are also topical enzymatic debriding agents available, but these work slowly and can also be painful in sensate patients.

The most effective debriding agent of all is to apply maggots to the wound. Thirty maggots have the ability to consume up to 1 gram of tissue per day, with the added benefit of consuming only necrotic tissue and bacteria. They leave all viable tissue intact. Maggots are relatively painless and are effective locally against antibiotic-resistant organisms. However, cooperation from both the patient and hospital staff is necessary for their use.

Post-Debridement

For extensive infection, with or without necrosis, repeat debridement every 12–48 hours until the wound is free from clinical signs of infection. This aggressive approach is often the only chance to save the diffusely infected limb.

When the blood supply is adequate, progressive tissue necrosis after debridement usually represents lingering uncontrolled infection and indicates that further debridement is needed.

Summary

Debridement is key to enabling chronic wounds to go through the normal healing process. An aggressive approach is sometimes required to create a healing environment and avoid amputation. Never condemn a limb to amputation too quickly, even if the amounts of infection and necrosis require extensive debridement. Debride only the normal-looking tissue, since the remaining tissue will be used for the subsequent reconstruction. The debridement process may leave the foot and leg with what appears to be a formidable reconstructive challenge. However, with modern reconstructive techniques, a functional limb can often be fashioned. In addition, short foot amputations, such as the Lisfranc or Chopart amputations, are viable options for the appropriate patient with the appropriate accommodative footwear. If, despite the above, a functional foot that matches the realistic functional goals of the patient cannot be reconstructed, a below-the-knee amputation should be considered.

References

1. Broughton G 2nd, Janis JE, Attinger CE. The basic science of wound healing. *Plast Reconstr Surg* 2006;117(Suppl. 7):12S–34S

2. Sheehan P, Jones P, Giurini JM, et al. Percent change in wound area of diabetic foot ulcers over a 4-week period is a robust predictor of complete healing in a 12-week prospective trial. *Plast Reconstr Surg* 2006;117 (Suppl. 7):239S–244S

3. Mustoe TA, O'Shaughnessy KO, Kloeters O. Chronic wound pathogenesis and current treatment strategies: a unifying hypothesis. *Plast Reconstr Surg* 2006;117(Suppl. 7):35S–41S

4. Davis SC, Martinez L, Kirsner R. The diabetic foot: the importance of biofilms and wound bed preparation. *Curr Diab Rep* 2006;6:439–445

5. Harding KG, Moore K, Phillips TJ. Wound chronicity and fibroblast senescence: implications for treatment. *Int Wound J* 2005;2:364–368

6. Armstrong DG, Lavery LA, Nixon BP, Boulton AJ. It's not what you put on, but what you take off: techniques for debriding and off-loading the diabetic foot wound. *Clin Infect Dis* 2004;39(Suppl. 2):S92–S99

7. Attinger CE, Bulan E, Blume PA. Surgical debridement: the key to successful wound healing and reconstruction. *Clin Podiatr Med Surg* 2000;17:599–630

8. Attinger CE, Janes JE, Steinberg JS, et al. Clinical approach to wounds: debridement and wound bed preparation including the use of dressings and wound-healing adjuvants. *Plast Reconstr Surg* 2006;117(Suppl. 7): 72S–109S

9. Caselli A, Latini V, Lapenna A, et al. Transcutaneous oxygen tension monitoring after successful revascularization in diabetic patients with ischaemic foot ulcers. *Diabet Med* 2005;22:460–465

10. Lipsky BA, Berendt AR, Cornia PB, et al. 2012 Infectious Diseases Society of America clinical practice guideline for the diagnosis and treatment of diabetic foot infections. *Clin Infect Dis* 2012;54:e132–e173

7
Adjunctive Wound Therapies

Katherine Baquerizo Nole, MD[1]; Paul E. Banwell, BSc (Hon), MB, BS, FRCS[2];
Julia Escandon, MD[1]; and Robert Kirsner, MD, PhD[1]
*[1]Department of Dermatology, University of Miami College of Medicine, Miami,
FL, and [2]The Banwell Clinic, East Grinstead, U.K.*

Adjunctive therapies—the use of dressings and other wound-healing therapies—form an important component of the holistic management of the diabetic foot. They augment and optimize the outcome of complex diabetic foot problems, and clinicians should be comfortable with the range of modalities and therapies available. For the diabetic neuropathic foot ulcer (DNFU), along with optimal glucose control, debridement, and offloading, adjunctive therapies form a tetrad of treatment. Close liaison with all members of the multidisciplinary team is required throughout the process.

Adjunctive therapies are classified as either passive or active. Passive therapies include dressings that have various functions but do not actively modulate the wound-healing environment. By contrast, active therapies include treatments that pharmacologically, biologically, or physically modulate the wound environment. Clinical data suggest size reduction, typically 50% after 4 weeks of standard care, predicts wound healing at 12 weeks;[1] for this reason, current Wound Healing Society guidelines recommend reevaluation or change of therapy if at least 40% wound size reduction is not achieved after 4 weeks.[2]

Wound Bed Preparation

Wound bed preparation refers to debridement of the wound edge and bed with the goal of removing necrotic material, nonfunctional cells, and bacteria,

DOI: 10.2337/9781580405706.07

potentially including biofilms. The concept of wound bed preparation was developed to address the overall state of the wound and the steps necessary both to optimize the endogenous processes of healing and to prepare the wound to allow optimal efficacy of advanced or adjunctive therapy.[3]

Although there are no data from randomized controlled trials, secondary analysis from advanced therapy trials and a large retrospective study have shown that performing debridement more frequently has higher wound-closure rates than less frequent debridement.[4-6]

Passive Therapies

Dressings

In combination with mechanical debridement, dressings can assist in the cleansing and sloughing of chronic wounds. Their primary purpose is to maintain a moist wound environment, which is conducive to healing via promotion of epithelialization. In addition, they protect the wound from external infection and trauma and absorb exudate to prevent maceration (when appropriate)—without adhering to the wound. Although there are no high-quality data showing a benefit of modern dressings over gauze, they do offer certain advantages, including longer wear time, greater absorption capacity, and potentially less pain and trauma upon removal.[7] Additionally, because of the lower frequency of dressing changes and less nursing time, modern dressings can be more cost-effective than traditional dressings.[8]

Dressings are divided into the following broad groups (Table 7.1):

- Low-adherent dressings include Melolin, paraffin gauze–based products, and silicone-based products.
- Semipermeable films are permeable to gases and vapor but impermeable to liquids and bacteria. These dressings usually have an adhesive backing and provide a moist wound environment. They are usually not suitable for heavily exudative wounds.
- Hydrogels are composed of a starch polymer matrix; they swell to absorb moisture and exudates. They also promote autolysis of necrotic material and slough and hence are useful alternatives or adjuncts to sharp debridement.
- Alginate dressings are derived from seaweed. They contain calcium, which activates the clotting cascade when mixed with sodium within the wound. This dressing becomes gelatinous upon absorbing moisture and can absorb

~20 times their weight, making them an excellent option for highly exudative wounds.[9]

- Synthetic foams are generally used in concave wounds and can conform to cavities, thus eliminating any potential dead space. They are suitable for heavily exudative wounds.

Table 7.1 Indications for Different Dressings

Appearance of the Wound	Therapeutic Alternatives
Presence of black, dry, necrotic tissue	Hydrogel dressings
Presence of fibrin or moist necrotic tissue	Hydrocolloid dressings
	Hydrogel dressings, if little exudate
	Alginate dressings, if heavily exuding
Cavity wound	Alginate ribbon dressings
	Hydrocolloid gel dressings
	Hydrocellular or foam pad dressings
Heavily exuding wound	Alginate dressings
	"New generation" hydrocolloid, hydrocellular dressings
Granulating wound	Hydrocolloid dressings
	Hydrocellular dressings
	Hydrogel dressings
	Hydrofiber dressings
	Transparent films
Superficial wound	Hydrocolloid dressings
	Hydrocellular or foam dressings
	Hydrogel dressings
	Film dressings
	Tulle and interface dressings
Foul-smelling wound	Charcoal dressings
Infected wound	Alginate dressings
	Silver-based dressings
	Cadexomer iodine dressings
	Honey dressings

It is important to consider the following criteria when choosing dressings:

- Appearance of the wound: presence of necrosis, slough, granulation tissue, or epithelialization
- Exudate: viscosity and volume
- Appearance of the skin around the wound
- Depth
- Odor
- Patient compliance
- Patient allergies and intolerance of products previously used
- Cost

Active Therapies

Bioengineered Products

The development of skin substitutes heralded the first useful bioengineered products. These products were originally designed for the massive skin loss associated with burns, but additional applications have evolved. Currently, there are a number of cellular bioengineered skin equivalents; however, only two of these products have been approved by the U.S. Food and Drug Administration (FDA) for treating diabetic foot ulcers. The first is Apligraf® (Organogenesis, Canton, MA), a living allogeneic bilayered construct containing keratinocytes, fibroblasts, and bovine type I collagen. The second, Dermagraft® (Organogenesis), is a dermal equivalent that contains living allogeneic dermal fibroblasts grown on a degradable scaffold[10] (Table 7.2).

Cells from these skin substitutes often do not persist for a prolonged time but rather supply growth factors and cytokines to speed healing.

The cell-based products have the strongest evidence of efficacy.[11] Apligraf® is made up of a cultured, living dermis and subsequently cultured epidermis, for which cellular components are derived from neonatal foreskin. When applied weekly for up to 5 weeks and followed for 12 weeks, the addition of Apligraf to a regimen of debridement and removable offloading devices improved healing (56 vs. 38%, $P = 0.0042$) and reduced the incidence of osteomyelitis and lower-limb amputations.[12]

A human fibroblast–derived dermis, Dermagraft®, is an allogeneic living dermal equivalent. Initial studies supported the benefit of Dermagraft (51% of ulcers healed at 12 weeks with Dermagraft versus 32% with control;

Table 7.2 Examples of Cellular Bioengineered Skin Equivalents

Components	Trade Names	Type	Composition	Indications	FDA Regulation
Epidermal	Epicel™	Auto-graft	Keratinocytes expanded	Deep dermal or full-thickness burns ≥30%	Humanitarian device
	EpiDex™	Auto-graft	Keratinocytes expanded from ORS cells of hair follicles	NA	NA
	BioSeed-S	Auto-graft	Keratinocytes in fibrin sealant	NA	NA
Dermal	Derma-graft®	Allo-graft	Allogenic—neonatal foreskin fibroblasts in polyglactin suture	Diabetic foot ulcers	Approved
Bilayered	Apligraf®	Allo-graft	Allogenic—engineered neonatal foreskin keratinocytes and fibroblasts plus bovine collagen type I	Venous leg ulcers Diabetic foot ulcers	Approved

NA, not applicable; ORS, Outer root sheath.

$P < 0.05$)[13] and led to a pivotal trial and FDA approval, in which after 12 weeks, 30% of Dermagraft patients healed, compared with 18.3% of the control patients. Dermagraft-treated patients were 1.7 times more likely to have complete wound closure at any given time than control patients and had a lower rate of ulcer-related adverse events.[14] Currently, a clinical trial comparing cellular versus acellular matrix devices is ongoing.[15]

Topical Negative Pressure or Negative Pressure Wound Therapy (NPWT) Vacuum-Assisted Closure

Topical negative pressure, or negative pressure wound therapy (NPWT), has an important role in modulating the wound-healing environment. A physical, nonpharmacological method of actively stimulating granulation tissue formation, this therapy applies mechanical forces across the wound, thus improving local blood flow and reducing edema. Furthermore, NPWT removes wound exudate and reduces the bioburden of wounds. The data support its use as an adjunct after a significant surgical procedure such as debridement or large excisional debridement, since it seems in DNFU, NPWT increases wound closure by ~50%,[16] decreases major amputations in >80%,[17] and may be less costly ($52,830 versus $61,757) than both traditional and advanced dressings.[18]

Although most studies evaluated an electrically powered Vacuum-Assisted Closure (VAC) Therapy System (Kinetic Concepts, Inc., San Antonio, TX), a recent ultraportable mechanically powered device (Smart Negative Pressure [SNaP] Wound Care System; Spiracur, Sunnyvale, CA) has shown equal efficacy in terms of wound closure, wound size reduction, and adverse events.[19]

Growth Factors

Despite the great expectations for growth factors in DNFU, only platelet-derived growth factor (PDGF) has enough evidence to gain FDA approval. It is currently commercialized as Regranex (becaplermin; Smith and Nephew, Ft. Worth, TX), and it has been shown to modestly improve healing (50% healing using PDGF versus 35% healing using normal saline dressings at 20 weeks) in several randomized clinical trials.[20] In a review of randomized controlled trials (922 patients with DNFU), daily becaplermin gel showed a healing rate of 83% as an adjunct to standard care.[21]

Preliminary data showed an increased risk of malignancy, which led to the FDA black box warning; however, a more recent large matched cohort with follow-up up to 6 years did not show an association.[22] This product may not be economically feasible in all health care environments.[23]

Topical and intralesional application of epidermal growth factor also demonstrated improved healing of diabetic foot ulcers, but the trials were small, and the product is not commercially available.[24] Factors such as nerve and neurotrophic growth factors and improved delivery of growth factors continue to be evaluated.

Hyperbaric Oxygen

Hyperbaric oxygen therapy (HBOT) is a short-term, high-dose oxygen inhalation and diffusion therapy delivered through airways to blood and tissue at a pressure higher than 1 ATA (absolute atmosphere). In clinical practice, 1–2.5 ATA are usually used. HBOT is currently reimbursed by the Center for Medicare and Medicaid Services in the United States for the treatment of diabetic foot ulcers,[25] and limited evidence from small randomized controlled trials and prospective studies suggests its efficacy for both ischemic and nonischemic ulcers.[26] However, the largest cohort of nonischemic DNFUs (~6,300 individuals) did not show benefits in wound healing or amputation rates when compared to standard care, suggesting use in practice may not follow the same criteria for patient selection and/or the same duration and time of therapy.[27] The main complications include barotrauma, myopia, cataract, seizures, and hypoglycemia; the most common cause of fatality is fire accidents, but that is exceedingly rare.[25]

Electrical Stimulation

Electrical stimulation appears to increase local blood flow in patients with diabetes.[28] The application of electric current to wound tissue may additionally affect protein synthesis, cell migration, and bacterial growth[2] and probably improves protective sensation and postural stability.[29] Trials performed have methodological limitations, but a recent systematic review of five trials found that electrical stimulation was associated with a statistically significant increase in healing rate when compared to control or sham (odds ratio 2.83, $P = 0.002$).[30]

References

1. Sheehan P, Jones P, Caselli A, et al. Percent change in wound area of diabetic foot ulcers over a 4-week period is a robust predictor of complete healing in a 12-week prospective trial. *Diabetes Care* 2003;26:1879–1882

2. Steed D, Attinger C, Colaizzi T, et al. Guidelines for the treatment of diabetic ulcers. *Wound Repair Regen* 2006;14:680–692

3. Falanga V, Brem H, Ennis W, et al. Maintenance debridement in the treatment of difficult-to-heal chronic wounds: recommendations of an expert panel. *Ostomy Wound Manage* 2008;June(Suppl.):2–13

4. Steed DL, Donohoe D, Webster MW, Lindsley L. Effect of extensive debridement and treatment on the healing of diabetic foot ulcers. *J Am Coll Surg* 1996;183:61–64

5. Cardinal M, Eisenbud DE, Armstrong DG, et al. Serial surgical debridement: a retrospective study on clinical outcomes in chronic lower extremity wounds. *Wound Repair Regen* 2009;17:306–311

6. Wilcox JR, Carter MJ, Covington S. Frequency of debridements and time to heal: a retrospective cohort study of 312744 wounds. *JAMA Dermatol* 2013;149:1050–1058

7. Alavi A, Sibbald RG, Mayer D, et al. Diabetic foot ulcers: part II: management. *J Am Acad Dermatol* 2014;70:e1–e24

8. Lo SF, Chang CJ, Hu WY, et al. The effectiveness of silver-releasing dressings in the management of non-healing chronic wounds: a meta-analysis. *J Clin Nurs* 2009;18:716–728

9. Sackheim K, De Araujo T, Kirsner RS. Compression modalities and dressings: their use in venous ulcers. *Dermatol Ther* 2006;19:338–347

10. Bello Y, Falabella A, Eaglstein H. Tissue-engineered skin: current status in wound healing. *Am J Clin Dermatol* 2001;2:305–313

11. Buchberger B, Follmann M, Freyer D, et al. The evidence for the use of growth factors and active skin substitutes for the treatment of non-infected diabetic foot ulcers (DFU): a health technology assessment (HTA). *Exp Clin Endocrinol Diabetes* 2011;119:472–479

12. Veves A, Falanga V, Armstrong DG, Sabolinski ML; Apligraf Diabetic Foot Ulcer Study. Graftskin, a human skin equivalent, is effective in the management of noninfected neuropathic diabetic foot ulcers: a prospective randomized multicenter clinical trial. *Diabetes Care* 2001;24:290–295

13. Gentzkow GD, Jensen JL, Pollak RA, et al. Improved healing of diabetic foot ulcers after grafting with a living human dermal replacement. *Wounds* 1999;11:77–84

14. Marston WA, Hanft J, Norwood P, Pollak R; Dermagraft Diabetic Foot Ulcer Study Group. The efficacy and safety of Dermagraft in improving the healing of chronic diabetic foot ulcers: results of a prospective randomized trial. *Diabetes Care* 2003;26:1701–1705

15. Lev-Tov H, Li CS, Dahle S, Isseroff RR. Cellular versus acellular matrix devices in treatment of diabetic foot ulcers: study protocol for a comparative efficacy randomized controlled trial. *Trials* 2013;14:8

16. Dumville JC, Hinchliffe RJ, Cullum N, et al. Negative pressure wound therapy for treating foot wounds in people with diabetes mellitus. *Cochrane Database Syst Rev* 2013;10:CD010318

17. Zhang J, Hu ZC, Chen D, et al. Effectiveness and safety of negative pressure wound therapy for diabetic foot ulcers: a meta-analysis. *Plast Reconstr Surg* 2014;134:141–151

18. Flack S, Apelqvist J, Keith M, et al. An economic evaluation of VAC therapy compared with wound dressings in the treatment of diabetic foot ulcers. *J Wound Care* 2008;17:71–78

19. Armstrong DG, Marston RA, Reyzelman AM, Kirsner RS. Comparative effectiveness of mechanically and electrically powered negative pressure wound therapy devices: a multicenter randomized controlled trial. *Wound Repair Regen* 2012;20:332–341

20. Steed DL. Clinical evaluation of recombinant human platelet-derived growth factor for the treatment of lower extremity diabetic ulcers: Diabetic Ulcer Study Group. *J Vasc Surg* 1995;21:71–78

21. Smiell JM, Wieman TJ, Steed DL, et al. Efficacy and safety of becaplermin (recombinant human platelet-derived growth factor-BB) in patients with nonhealing, lower extremity diabetic ulcers: a combined analysis of four randomized studies. *Wound Repair Regen* 1999;7:335–346

22. Ziyadeh N, Fife D, Walker AM, et al. A matched cohort study of the risk of cancer in users of becaplermin. *Adv Skin Wound Care* 2011;24:31–39

23. Sibbald RG, Torrance G, Hux M, et al. Cost-effectiveness of becaplermin for nonhealing neuropathic diabetic foot ulcers. *Ostomy Wound Manage* 2003;49:76–84

24. Gomez-Villa R, Aguilar-Rebolledo F, Lozano-Platonoff A, et al. Efficacy of intralesional recombinant human epidermal growth factor in diabetic foot ulcers in Mexican patients: a randomized double-blinded controlled trial. *Wound Repair Regen* 2014;22:497–503

25. Löndahl M. Hyperbaric oxygen therapy as adjunctive treatment of diabetic foot ulcers. *Med Clin North Am* 2013;97:957–980

26. Kranke P, Bennett M, Roeckl-Wiedmann I, Debus S. Hyperbaric oxygen therapy for chronic wounds. *Cochrane Database Syst Rev* 2004;2:CD004123

27. Margolis DJ, Gupta J, Hoffstad O, et al. Lack of effectiveness of hyperbaric oxygen therapy for the treatment of diabetic foot ulcer and the prevention of amputation: a cohort study. *Diabetes Care* 2013;36:1961–1966

28. Baker LL, Chambers R, DeMuth SK, Villar F. Effects of electrical stimulation on wound healing in patients with diabetic ulcers. *Diabetes Care* 1997;20:405–412

29. Najafi B, Crews RT, Wrobel JS. A novel plantar stimulation technology for improving protective sensation and postural control in patients with diabetic peripheral neuropathy: a double-blinded, randomized study. *Gerontology* 2013;59:473–480

30. Kwan RL, Cheing GL, Vong SK, Lo SK. Electrophysical therapy for managing diabetic foot ulcers: a systematic review. *Int Wound J* 2013; 10:121–131

Suggested Readings

Cavorsi J, Vicari F, Wirthlin DJ, et al. Best-practice algorithms for the use of a bilayered living cell therapy (Apligraf) in the treatment of lower-extremity ulcers. *Wound Repair Regen* 2006;14:102–109

8
Dressings and Local Wound Care for People with Diabetic Foot Wounds

R. Gary Sibbald, MD, FRCPC (Med Derm), FAAD, MACP, MEd, FAPWCA, DSc (Hons)[1]; James Elliott, MMSc, BSc[2]; and Elizabeth A. Ayello, PhD, RN, ACNS-BC, CWON, ETN, MAPWCA, FAAN[3]

[1]*Department of Medicine, Division of Dermatology, University of Toronto College of Medicine, Toronto, Canada;* [2]*Independent Researcher, Toronto, Canada; and* [3]*The John A. Hartford Institute for Geriatric Nursing, New York, NY*

As with all chronic wounds, wound bed preparation (WBP) principles (Fig. 8.1) apply to the treatment of diabetic foot wounds.[1] Care is best achieved when clinician assessment of the wound is coupled with a process to mutually incorporate patient/family-centered concerns. Selecting the most appropriate dressing, a component of local wound care within the WBP model, can be a complex process. In this chapter, key aspects of the WBP model and its application to people with diabetic foot wounds and their local wound care are explored.

Treating the Cause of Diabetic Foot Wounds

There are three important components when assessing a person with a diabetic foot wound. These components are identified with the mnemonic VIP:

- **V**ascular supply: A palpable foot pulse, an ankle brachial pressure index >0.5, or a toe pressure >55 mmHg should be present; if not, the patient needs vascular assessment for bypass or dilation.
- **I**nfection: Infection of the deep and surrounding tissue with any three of the seven clinical signs identified by the mnemonic STONEES

DOI: 10.2337/9781580405706.08

Wound Bed Preparation 2015

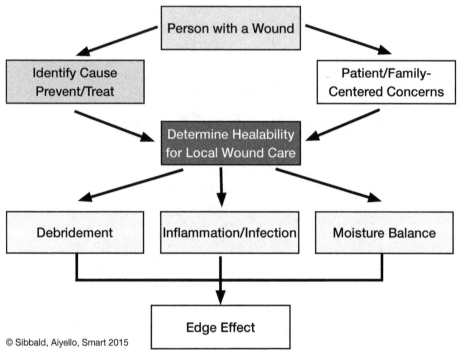

© Sibbald, Aiyello, Smart 2015

Figure 8.1—Wound bed preparation 2015

requires systemic antimicrobial agents. These seven clinical STONEES signs are:

1. **S**ize of wound expanding
2. **T**emperature increase with infrared thermometry
3. **O**s = Latin for bone: probing or exposed bone
4. **N**ew or satellite areas of breakdown
5. **E**rythema/**E**dema = cellulitis of surrounding skin
6. **S**mell = the presence of gram negatives or anaerobic organisms[2]

- **Pressure:** There is a need for plantar pressure redistribution with orthotics, shoes, or special devices. A callus means increased pressure. A blister signifies friction or shear between the footwear and the patient.

Patient-Centered Concerns

It is paramount to consider the whole patient before the hole in the patient. Assess for pain, barriers to activities of everyday living, depression, anxiety, and other unaddressed patient-centered concerns. Bear in mind the importance of adequate blood glucose control; healing delay is directly correlated with elevated HbA_{1c} in people with diabetes.[3] Further, patients may not display signs of infection when HbA_{1c} is >12%. Adequate blood flow is necessary for wound healing. Because each cigarette diminishes circulation for 1 hour, it is worthwhile to explore tobacco-cessation strategies with patients who smoke.

Wound-associated pain is often the most important patient concern.[4] It can occur at dressing change, with debridement, or from the wound etiology between dressing changes. Wound-associated pain can be divided into two broad categories: nociceptive pain (i.e., stimulus-dependent), often described as gnawing, aching, tender, or throbbing, and neuropathic pain (i.e., non–stimulus-dependent), often described as burning, stinging, shooting, or stabbing.

Determine Healability

Based on clinician assessment of the wound and the patient's ability to adhere to a proposed treatment plan, "healability" (or the ability of the wound to heal) can be determined.[1] The three classes of a wound pertaining to healability are:

1. Healable: Treatment of the cause and enough blood supply to heal
2. Maintenance: Is not healable, since the patient cannot adhere to the plan of care or health system issues prevent a care plan that could lead to healing
3. Non-healable: The cause cannot be corrected (e.g., non-bypassable or dilatable vessels in an ischemic foot)

Local Wound Care

The location, area (length multiplied by widest width at right angles), and depth of the ulcer, in addition to the type and amount of exudate should be documented at every visit. Assessment for infection should be determined by identifying 3 of the 7 STONEES criteria, including the measurement of peri-wound skin temperature with an infrared thermometer.[5] Dressing choices should be determined by the healability of the diabetic foot ulcer and the need for debridement, infection or inflammation control, and moisture balance. Little high-quality evidence exists to guide dressing choices in clinical practice.[6] Most settings use expert knowledge, clinical experience, and patient preference to match the form and function of available dressings to wound characteristics. Effective dressing selection and local wound care planning involve the perspectives of the entire interprofessional team.[7]

Case Vignette 1

Dr. Jones, a podiatrist, works at an outpatient wound center. Dressings in this setting are incident to the procedure performed (i.e., the clinic cannot charge extra for the dressings applied at a wound center visit). Dr. Jones usually chooses an alginate rope as the primary dressing post-debridement based on the following performance parameters (modified from Cockbill and Turner[8]):

- *Hemostatic properties*: Dressing donates calcium for the hemostatic process on the skin surface. It also accepts sodium, converting the dressing from a fiber to a hydrogel for moist interactive healing. This process prevents development of a proinflammatory crust and facilitates the wound moving from the inflammatory to the proliferative stage.
- *Gelling*: A moist wound-healing environment causes the dressing to bio-absorb. If there are fibers that are not hydrated, then the exudate is not sufficient to completely resorb the dressing. If there is minimal exudate, a less absorptive dressing should be substituted or the dressing wear time can be increased with a more absorptive dressing.
- *Cost-effectiveness*: Alginate dressings are a relatively affordable option.
- *Compatibility with silver*: This dressing can be combined with silver if antimicrobial properties are required. There should be three or more signs of critical colonization for an antimicrobial dressing. Use the **NERDS** mnemonic for signs of critical colonization: **N**on-healing: the wound does not decrease in size over 2–4 weeks; increased **E**xudate; **R**ed friable granulation instead of firm pink tissue; **D**ebris or dead tissue on the wound surface; and **S**mell, usually from gram-negative or anaerobic organisms.[2] Silver needs to be ionized in an aqueous environment to be active. If there is a dry surface, silver is not the correct antimicrobial choice.

Dressings Within the Overall Plan of Care

After the wound bed is prepared and cleansed, a dressing that fits within the overall plan of care must be chosen. Four questions the clinician should consider are:

1. What is the underlying wound etiology (e.g., pressure, neuropathic, neuroischemic, or ischemic components)?
2. Is the wound healable, maintenance, or non-healable?
3. Is the wound colonized, critically colonized, or infected?[2,9]
4. Is the plan of care aggressive, maintenance, or palliative?

Dressing selection is just one piece of the puzzle; dressings alone will not promote healing unless the underlying cause of the wound is addressed. Nonetheless, careful attention to dressing selection can reduce pain, optimize the wound environment for healing, and improve quality of life. On the other hand, inappropriate dressing selection can cause wounds to deteriorate with:

- Wound margin maceration if there is inadequate exudate management
- Skin stripping, increasing the risk of infection
- Increased local pressure, causing callus formation
- Friction and shear, leading to blisters, erosions, increased pain, and slower healing.

An inappropriate dressing selection can cause delayed healing with extra cost to the patient and health system. For healable wounds, dressings should maintain a moist healing environment (moisture balance), whereas for a maintenance or non-healable wound, moisture reduction is required. Clinicians must reevaluate the plan of care frequently, since local wound conditions can often change, even on a daily basis.

Case Vignette 2

Mary Silver, a 78-year-old diabetes patient, developed a stage 4 pressure ulcer of the left heel after a fall that fractured her right hip and caused an open reduction internal fixation of the femur. The eschar was debrided, and there was a red wound base. Mrs. Silver was then transferred to a long-term care facility for rehabilitation. During wound rounds, the hospital wound team evaluated the situation, talked to Mrs. Silver, and identified the need for the following:

- Moist wound-healing environment to promote granulation tissue formation
- Non-bulky dressing that will accommodate her diabetic footwear without causing pressure

• Waterproof dressing for daily bathing and hygiene (patient preference)

The team recommends that the following dressing procedure be used at the long-term care facility:

• Cleanse wound with normal saline
• Apply very thin layer of amorphous hydrogel to wound base
• Cover with an adhesive film dressing
• Change Monday, Wednesday, and Friday and as needed

Clinical Goals

Identifying the clinical goal(s) for a dressing helps to focus dressing selection from the myriad of categories available. Clinical goals for dressings include:

• Pain management
• Debridement
• Bioburden control (critical colonization, surface bacterial damage)
• Exudate management
• Moisture balance
• Protecting wound margins
• Odor control

Other essential considerations include the following:

• Access
• Context of care
• Insurance coverage/allowable products
• Patient preference

Dressing Formularies

A typical dressing formulary for a facility might include 10–20 different dressing options.[10] Table 8.1 gives an example of a typical dressing formulary by generic category with properties and other comments.

Case Vignette 3

Tim Ott is a 53-year-old male who has had type 2 diabetes for over 20 years. Over the last month, he noted that his blood glucose was erratic and he had developed an ulcer over a previously callused area on his left first metatarsal

Table 8.1 Typical Dressing Formulary by Generic Category

Dressing	Properties	Autolytic Debridement	Antibacterial Versions Available	Moisture Balance
Superabsorbent	Diaper technology for maximum absorbency	No	No	Creates a moisture lock, wicking excess exudate away from the wound surface
Foam	Polyurethane with uniform or variable pore sizes. Wound surface: nonadhesive, adhesive, silicone Backing often polyurethane film	No, except for polyvinyl alcohol forms including methylene blue/ crystal violet foam formulation	Yes, with silver plus moist surface	Moisture exchange, if overlapping on the wound margin, can cause periwound maceration
Hydrofiber	Carboxymethylcellulose (CMC) that binds moisture to surface Not bio-resorbable	No, or minor	Yes, with silver plus moist surface	Fluid lock but lower absorbency and leaves fluid close to wound
Calcium alginate	Hemostasis (post-debridement) Bio-resorbable Rope (packing) or wafer	Yes, with formation of the hydrogel when sodium replaces calcium	Yes, with silver plus moist surface	Binds water on the surface with formation of a hydrogel
Hydrogel	70–90% water with gelling agent (saline, propylene glycol, glycerin hydrocolloid = CMC) Amorphous and sheet forms	Yes, with hard eschar breakdown facilitated by scoring the wound (linear groves without bleeding)	Yes, with silver or a low gel pH (glycerin/ CMC)	Donates water to hydrate a wound promoting cellular function plus autolytic debridement
Hydrocolloid	Water-loving (carboxyl) and repelling (methylcellulose) with adhesive and additives plus a backing	Yes, with the carboxyl terminal as well as gelatin/ pectin additives	Yes, with low pH plus occlusion	Some absorbency with a long wear time

Table 8.1 Typical Dressing Formulary by Generic Category *(continued)*

Dressing	Properties	Autolytic Debridement	Antibacterial Versions Available	Moisture Balance
Transparent film	Used as protectant or secondary dressing Accumulated moisture or loss of seal requires changing	Yes, trapped moisture can facilitate autolytic debridement but may be a nidus for infection	Yes, with silver plus moist surface	Traps minimal moisture
Nonadherent gauze	Smooth surface to protect wound or act as a secondary dressing	No	Yes, with silver plus moist surface	No, with evaporation can stick to the wound causing pain plus trauma on removal
Contact layer	A nonadherent layer used for wound protection under a secondary dressing or bandage	No	Yes, with silver plus moist surface	No
Composite	A combination of two dressing categories, often a central absorbent island attached to an adhesive backing	Only if the island dressing is an autolytic debriding agent	Yes, with silver plus moist surface	Yes, with absorptive surface but can lead to wound dehydration
Antiseptic	Agents that have broad-spectrum antimicrobial action in a dry environment (povidone iodine, chlorhexidine) Tissue toxicity must be balanced with antimicrobial effect	No, unless combined with cadexomer or other agent	Yes, unlikely to cause resistance	No, unless combined with other agents

Two excellent online dressing resources are available to help build a dressing formulary by generic category: Wound Source (Kestrel Health, U.S.), www.woundsource.com, and World Wide Wounds (U.K.), www.worldwidewounds.com.

head. The ulcer was discharging pus, and he has pain in the foot even though he has a loss of protective sensation.

Clinical assessment revealed clawed toes on the left foot associated with an ulcer beneath the first metatarsal head of the foot, measuring 2 × 2 cm. There was a surrounding 3+ out of 4 hyperkeratotic callus, with the ulcer probing to bone. The ulcer base contained bright red friable granulation with a thick pustular-purulent discharge. The skin surface temperature with an infrared thermometer was 8°F warmer than the mirror-image second metatarsal head on the right foot. X-ray revealed active osteomyelitis. A difference of 3°F or higher is a clinical sign of infection. There was probing to bone and a purulent exudate (3 of the 7 STONEES signs).

The palpable pulse indicated adequate vascular supply for healing. Mr. Ott was started on systemic antimicrobial therapy covering gram-positives, gram-negatives, and anaerobic organisms. His ulcer was initially packed with povidone iodine gauze, since antibacterial action at this stage was more important than tissue toxicity. This treatment continued until the deep tissue infection was under control. The dressing was then changed to a cadexomer iodine and later to crystal violet/methylene blue foam to support moist interactive healing, autolytic debridement, and surface critical colonization. Plantar pressure redistribution was accomplished with a pneumatic walker made irremovable with a fiberglass external bandage. The hyperkeratotic callus was surgically debrided, and the surface of the wound was cleaned with a curette to a lightly bleeding wound surface every 1–2 weeks, until complete wound healing was accomplished in 10 weeks.

Evidence-Informed Dressing Selection

Current consensus for healable wounds recommends dressings that maintain a moist wound-healing environment, manage exudate, control bioburden, and minimize pain with the potential to improve wound healing outcomes.[10,11] Wet-to-dry gauze dressings, a method of mechanical debridement, are less desirable because of trauma on removal and the excess nursing time required for daily dressing changes compared to the longer wear time associated with more modern moist wound dressings.

In the United States, the Centers for Medicare and Medicaid Services (CMS) gives specific guidance on how to classify, in long-term care, if a wound is a pressure ulcer or a diabetic foot ulcer (on MDS 3.0 section M). If there is a

Table 8.2 Antimicrobial Dressings for Healable Diabetic Foot Ulcers

Antimicrobial Component	Moisture Balance Component	Comments and Precautions
Silver: antiinflammatory	Foam, alginate, hydrofibers, hydrogel	• Needs moisture to be ionized and needs an active antimicrobial • Avoid close contact with zinc, petrolatum
Iodine: proinflammatory	Cadexomer	• Use with caution if thyroid disease is present
PHMB (polyhexamethyl-enebiguanide): non-release, neutral	Foam	• Cidal due to destruction of the cell wall
Crystal violet/methylene blue: mild release, low toxicity	Foam	• Polyvinyl alcohol foam facilitates autolytic debridement

wound on the lower extremity, for example, the heel in a person with diabetes, and the primary etiology is pressure, then the CMS RAI manual directs that this wound should be coded as a pressure ulcer (section M0300) and not a diabetic foot ulcer (www.cms.gov). Also visit http://www.cms.gov/Medicare/Quality-Initiatives-Patient-Assessment-Instruments/NursingHomeQuality-Inits/MDS30RAIManual.html for more information. If a wound is diabetes-related, it is coded in section 1040B.

Finally, consideration must be given to regulatory requirements such as these from CMS:

- For Medicare Part B patients, the Surgical Dressing Policy (2079), available on the Durable Medical Equipment (DME) Region A, B, C, and D websites.
- For long-term care facilities, F-Tag 314 Pressure Ulcer Guidance for Surveyors: http://www.annalsoflongtermcare.com/attachments/5552.pdf
- For long-term care facilities and long-term acute care hospitals (LTCHs), CMS MDS 3.0 section M skin conditions: http://www.cms.gov/Medi-

care/Quality-Initiatives-Patient-Assessment-Instruments/Nursing-HomeQualityInits/MDS30RAIManual.html
- For inpatient rehabilitation CMS IRF-RAI instrument: http://www.cms.gov/Medicare/Medicare-Fee-for-Service-Payment/InpatientRehab-FacPPS/IRFPAI.html
- For the LTCH training manual: http://www.cms.gov/Medicare/Quality-Initiatives-Patient-Assessment-Instruments/LTCH-Quality-Reporting/LTCH-Quality-Reporting-Training.html

Numerous clinical practice guidelines recommend dressing selection and should be consulted when dressing formularies are developed. Selected evidence-informed guidelines include the following:

For diabetic foot wounds:

- American Diabetes Association. Standards of medical care in diabetes—2013. *Diabetes Care* 2013;36(Suppl. 1):S11–S66
- American Diabetes Association. Consensus Development Conference on Diabetic Foot Wound Care: 7–8 April 1999, Boston, Massachusetts. *Diabetes Care* 1999;22:1354–1360
- International Best Practice Guidelines: Wound Management in Diabetic Foot Ulcers. Wounds International, 2013: www.woundsinternational.com
- Bakker K, Apelqvist J, Schaper NC, on behalf of the International Working Group on the Diabetic Foot Editorial Board. Practical guidelines on the management and prevention of the diabetic foot 2011. *Diabetes Metab Res Rev* 2012;28:225–231
- World Union of Wound Healing Societies: www.woundpedia.com
- Crawford PE, Fields-Varnado M; WOCN Society. Guideline for the management of wounds in patients with lower-extremity neuropathic disease: an executive summary. *J Wound Ostomy Continence Nurs* 2013;40:34–45: www.wocn.org

For pressure ulcers:

- American Medical Directors Association. Clinical practice guidelines for pressure ulcers, 2008; reaffirmed in 2013: www.amda.com
- National Pressure Ulcer Advisory Panel/European Pressure Ulcer Advisory Panel/Pan Pacific Pressure Injury Alliance. Pressure ulcer prevention and treatment guideline, 2014: www.npuap.org and www.epuap.org

- World Union of Wound Healing Societies: www.woundpedia.com
- Wound Healing Society guidelines for the treatment of pressure ulcers, 2006: www.whs.org
- Wound, Ostomy, and Continence Nurses Society guidelines for the prevention and management of pressure ulcers, 2010: www.wocn.org

Summary

People with diabetic foot wounds should receive holistic care that treats the cause and patient-centered concerns. These care elements need to be addressed before the issues of local wound care, since dressings alone will not promote healing unless the underlying cause is addressed. Careful attention to dressing selection has many benefits, including improved patient healing outcomes, reduced pain, enhanced quality of life, and cost-effective care. The plan of care has a stronger foundation when an interprofessional team is involved in holistic care, including local wound care and dressing selection. Incorporating patient preferences within the context of evidence-informed practice is more likely to promote patient adherence and the successful healing of diabetic foot wounds. Clinicians must often reevaluate plans of care frequently as local wound conditions can change.

Acknowledgment

We gratefully acknowledge the contributions of Diane L. Krasner, PhD, RN, CWCN, CWS, BCLNC, FAAN, to the previous edition of this chapter.

References

1. Sibbald RG, Goodman L, Woo KY, et al. Special considerations in wound bed preparation 2011: an update. *Adv Skin Wound Care* 2011;24:415–436

2. Woo KY, Sibbald RG. A cross-sectional validation study of using NERDS and STONEES to assess bacterial burden. *Ostomy Wound Manage* 2009;55:40–48

3. Christmas A, Selvin E, Margolis D, et al. Hemoglobin A1c predicts healing rate in diabetic wounds. *J Invest Dermatol* 2011;131:2121–2127

4. Woo KY, Abbott LK, Librach L. Evidence-based approach to manage persistent wound-related pain: *Curr Opin Support Palliat Care* 2013;7:86–94

5. Sibbald RG, Mufti A, Armstrong DG. Infrared skin thermometry: an under-utilized cost-effective tool for routine wound care practice and patient high-risk diabetic foot self-monitoring. *Adv Skin Wound Care* 2015;28;37–44

6. Dumville JC, Deshpande S, O'Meara S, Speak K. Foam dressings for healing diabetic foot ulcers. In *Cochrane Database of Systematic Reviews.* The Cochrane Collaboration, Ed. Chichester, U.K., John Wiley & Sons, 2013. http://doi.wiley.com/10.1002/14651858.CD009111.pub3

7. Krasner D, Rodeheaver GT, Sibbald RG. Interprofessional wound caring. In *Chronic Wound Care: A Clinical Source Book for Healthcare Professionals.* 4th ed. Krasner DL, Rodeheaver GT, Sibbald RG, Eds. Malvern, PA, HMP Communications, 2007, p. 3–9

8. Cockbill SME, Turner TD. The development of wound management products. In *Chronic Wound Care: A Clinical Source Book for Healthcare Professionals.* 4th ed. Krasner DL, Rodeheaver GT, Sibbald RG, Eds. Malvern, PA, HMP Communications, 2007, p. 233–248

9. Sibbald RG, Woo K, Ayello EA. Increased bacterial burden and infection: the story of NERDS and STONES. *Adv Skin Wound Care* 2006;19:447–461

10. Broussard CL. Dressing decisions. In *Chronic Wound Care: A Clinical Source Book for Healthcare Professionals.* 4th ed. Krasner DL, Rodeheaver GT, Sibbald RG, Eds. Malvern, PA, HMP Communications, 2007, p. 249–262

11. Jones V, Harding K. Moist wound healing: optimizing the wound environment. In *Chronic Wound Care: A Clinical Source Book for Healthcare Professionals.* 4th ed. Krasner DL, Rodeheaver GT, Sibbald RG, Eds. Malvern, PA, HMP Communications, 2007, p. 199–204

Suggested Readings

Sibbald RG, Orsted HL, Coutts PM, Keast DH. Best practice recommendations for preparing the wound bed: update 2006. *Advances Skin Wound Care* 2007;20:390–405

Sibbald RG, Williamson D, Orsted HL, et al. Preparing the wound bed: debridement, bacterial balance, and moisture balance. *Ostomy Wound Manage* 2000;46:14–37

9
The Diabetic Charcot Foot: Recognition, Evaluation, and Management

Lee C. Rogers, DPM[1]; Robert G. Frykberg, DPM, MPH[2]; and Lee J. Sanders, DPM[3]
[1]*Amputation Prevention Centers of America, Los Angeles, CA;* [2]*Department of Veterans Affairs, Phoenix, AZ; and* [3]*Department of Veterans Affairs, Lebanon, PA*

Diabetes is the leading cause of neuropathic osteoarthropathy (aka, Charcot's joint disease, Charcot neuroarthropathy, Charcot's arthropathy, diabetic neuropathic osteoarthropathy, and the Charcot foot), a rare and potentially disabling condition affecting the foot and ankle.[1] Jean-Martin Charcot (1825–1893) is properly credited with the description of a unique group of arthropathies affecting the long bones and joints of the knee, hip, and shoulder in patients with tabes dorsalis (neurosyphilis).[2,3] However, it was Herbert W. Page (1845–1926), an English surgeon, who was the first to chronicle involvement of the small bones and joints of the foot and ankle in a patient with tabes dorsalis.[4] Page provided the earliest description of the rocker-bottom foot deformity associated with this malady. He advocated for heightened awareness, recognition, and documentation of this arthropathy. In 1883, Jean-Martin Charcot and Charles Féré[5] published their first investigation of this condition, a small case series, in which they described their observations of the bone and joint conditions affecting the feet of patients with tabes dorsalis (pied tabétique). Of the five case observations discussed in this chapter, pattern II was the incident case presented by Herbert W. Page in 1881 at the International Medical Congress in London.[5] The condition described by Charcot and Féré as pied tabétique has come to be known as the Charcot foot.

DOI: 10.2337/9781580405706.09

Symptoms

Early symptoms of the Charcot foot can be subtle, with mild swelling, redness, and a localized increase in the skin temperature of the foot and ankle, so the condition often goes unrecognized. Sometimes, the foot suddenly and unexpectedly collapses, with fractures, dislocations, and ulceration. Remarkably, these destructive events occur in the absence of major trauma. Even after the condition has matured, the bone and joint changes may resemble osteomyelitis, further confusing the diagnosis.

Unfortunately, recognition and treatment of the Charcot foot remain significant problems and the precise pathogenesis of the condition is an enigma. Clinicians must therefore be watchful for it, especially in that subset of diabetic patients who are considered to be at high risk for developing the condition. These patients typically have a long history of diabetes (10–15 years' duration) and demonstrate evidence of sensory-motor-autonomic neuropathy. The clinical picture is characterized by loss of protective sensation, lack of deep tendon reflexes, diminished or absent vibratory sensation, and the presence of palpable (often bounding) pedal pulses. Autonomic neuropathy can be elicited by testing for heart rate variability with deep breathing This normal physiologic arrhythmia is often absent in individuals with Charcot foot.[6] Before the acute onset of neuropathic osteoarthropathy, patients may experience painful sensory neuropathy characterized by lancinating pains, like a shower of electric needles, of short duration but recurrent throughout the day.[1] Characteristics include the following:

- The acute Charcot foot may mimic cellulitis, acute gouty arthritis, or thrombophlebitis. In earlier presentations, it may be indistinguishable from osteoarthritis or osteomyelitis.
- Pain may be absent or minimal, which is surprising to most clinicians, considering the extensive bone and joint pathology seen in some cases.
- Radiographs may initially appear unremarkable. Early radiographic findings can be absent or so subtle that they are easily missed by the untrained eye. This result was previously categorized as "stage 0" Charcot foot, since the acute destructive process has not yet commenced.[7] A minimally displaced fracture at the base of the second metatarsal, which may precede collapse of the tarsometatarsal joints (Fig. 9.1), is especially likely to be missed. A negative report can lead the clinician to mistakenly treat the condition as an infection, gout, or deep vein thrombosis and to lose valu-

able time. This error can also become a litigious issue for the clinician and the radiologist. Whenever possible, clinicians should view the radiographs themselves and not rely solely on the radiologist's interpretation.

- Early identification of Charcot's joint disease is crucial, with immediate rest, immobilization, and offloading recommended. Until the diagnosis is safely ruled out, err on the side of early aggressive treatment, with immobilization and offloading. A cavalier watch-and-wait approach could be disastrous.

- For individuals at high risk, patient education is essential. Discuss the implications of sensory loss, the signs and symptoms of diabetic neuropathic osteoarthropathy, the importance of therapeutic footwear, and the need for preventive foot care.

Prevalence and Risk Factors

The prevalence of diagnosed neuropathic osteoarthropathy associated with diabetes has been reported to be from 0.08 to 13%.[8] The incidence is believed to be <1%. Unfortunately, there are no high-quality epidemiologic studies of the diabetic Charcot foot because of the lack of a clear definition and confirmatory diagnostic tests for this condition. A prospective study of 1,666 patients from a disease management program in Texas found the incidence of Charcot arthropathy to be 8.5/1,000 per year.[9] A study of radiographic abnormalities in the feet of neuropathic diabetic subjects revealed that 9% of the patients had evidence of Charcot's joint disease.[10] The true incidence of osteoarthropathy in diabetes is limited by few prospective or population-based studies. Available data are mainly based on retrospective studies of small single-center cohorts. In addition, because many cases go undetected, especially in the early stages, the prevalence has probably been underestimated. However, reported cases of the diabetic Charcot foot appear to be on the rise as a result of increased awareness of its signs and symptoms.

The primary risk factors for the Charcot foot are the presence of dense peripheral sensory neuropathy and a history of preceding trauma, often minor in nature. A careful history will often reveal a precipitating event, such as a minor ankle sprain or contusion that preceded collapse of the foot. Foot and ankle deformities, limited joint mobility (such as limited ankle joint dorsiflexion caused by contracture and decreased elasticity of the Achilles tendon), faulty biomechanics, or surgical trauma can also trigger Charcot's joint disease.[1]

Clinicians must be aware that the Charcot foot is a progressive condition characterized by joint dislocation, pathologic fractures, and collapse of the foot and ankle. Ultimately, this condition can lead to debilitating deformity, instability of the foot and ankle, ulceration, infection, and amputation.

Etiology of Neuropathic Osteoarthropathy

Charcot's joint disease is most likely the result of the combined effects of neurovascular and neurotraumatic etiologies.[11] Minor injury of a neuropathic limb can precipitate the development of an active Charcot foot. Autonomic nervous system dysfunction has also been associated with neuropathic osteoarthropathy.

A neurally initiated vascular reflex leading to increased peripheral blood flow and active bone resorption may be another important etiologic factor. Autonomic neuropathy with loss of vasomotor control and increased peripheral blood flow to the bone, coupled with an inflammatory hyperemia of the soft tissues, results in resorption and weakening of bone. Atrophic osteopenic bone is easily fractured or fragmented. Sensory neuropathy renders the patient unaware of precipitating injuries and the osseous destruction taking place during unrestricted physical activities. A vicious cycle develops in which the patient continues to walk on the injured foot, thereby causing further damage.

There are current investigations into the putative roles of proinflammatory cytokines (tumor necrosis factor [TNF]-α, interleukin [IL]-1, and IL-6) and the RANKL (receptor activator for nuclear factor Kβ [RANK] ligand)/RANK/ OPG (osteoprotegerin) signaling pathway in the development of osteoclastogenesis and perpetuation of inflammation in the acute Charcot foot.[12,13] Recent evidence also suggests that single nucleotide polymorphisms for the *OPG* gene might play a role in determining susceptibility for this disorder.[14]

Diagnosis of the Acute Charcot Foot

Diagnosis of the acute Charcot foot requires a detailed clinical history, physical examination, and radiographic studies, with a high index of suspicion for the disease in a high-risk population of individuals with diabetes, peripheral neuropathy, and a well-vascularized foot. The diagnostic delay averages 29 weeks,[15] and the condition is commonly misdiagnosed in the general clinic or emergency room setting.[16] Nearly all reports confirm the role of trauma in initiating the evolution of Charcot's joint disease. Physical findings include unilateral swelling of the foot or ankle, elevated skin temperature compared with the contralateral limb, erythema, palpable bounding pedal pulses, and peripheral sensory neuropathy with loss of protective sensation. Neuropathy is an absolute requirement for development of Charcot's joint disease. Associated risk factors include diminished bone mineral density, localized osteopenia, and history of pancreas-kidney transplantation. Early radiographic findings may be negative or very subtle. Positive findings may reveal bone resorption (typically in the forefoot), diastasis (>2 mm separation at the bases of the first and second metatarsal bone), subluxation/dislocation (typically at the tarsometatarsal, naviculocuneiform, or midtarsal joints), or fracture(s). Look carefully at the base of the second metatarsal (Fig. 9.1).

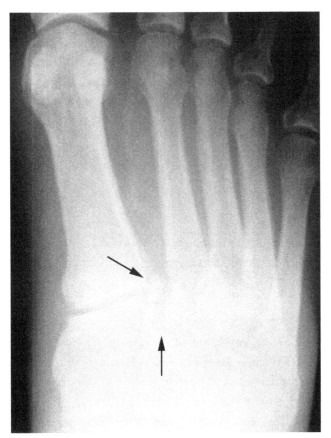

Figure 9.1—Early presentation of the Charcot foot with subtle findings at the tarsometatarsal joints (pattern II). Note the displaced fracture at the base of the second metatarsal bone with >2 mm separation at the bases of the first and second metatarsal bones.

Radiographs of the opposite foot are helpful for comparison. Bilateral involvement has been reported to occur in 5.9–39.3% of cases. Usually, no further imaging studies are needed to establish the diagnosis, since radiographs and clinical features are often sufficient.

Laboratory studies ordered for the acute Charcot foot typically reveal normal white blood cell count, normal C-reactive protein, normal serum uric acid, negative Duplex scan, and positive bone scan (nonspecific). However, the caveat is that the presence of ulceration and soft tissue infection may further confuse the diagnosis, making it difficult to differentiate between acute neuropathic osteoarthropathy (noninfective bone disease) and osteomyelitis. Ulcers that probe to bone are highly suggestive of osteomyelitis.

A bone biopsy can be of use if the diagnosis remains equivocal after routine laboratory testing and imaging. Core needle bone biopsy is the most specific test to distinguish between osteomyelitis and osteoarthropathy. Characteristic histological findings associated with neuropathic osteoarthropathy include the following:

- Erosion of articular cartilage
- Active resorption of bone with thin, widely spaced trabeculae
- Increased vascularity
- New bone formation
- Remodeling

When the ankle joint is involved, there is a striking pathologic feature of bone and cartilage debris (detritus) ground into the synovial tissue and articular cartilage.

Imaging of the Charcot Foot

Imaging modalities are important in diagnosing Charcot foot and differentiating it from other bone disorders. Plain film radiography is still the most useful modality for diagnosis and prognosticating. The characteristic changes on X-ray depend on the stage in which the Charcot joint appears. Early in the pathologic process, there may be some lysis in the periarticular areas, but occasionally there are no changes visible. As the disease progresses, deformity, including joint subluxations, dislocation, or frank fractures, may be visible. Osteomyelitis is another common bone condition afflicting the feet of individuals with diabetes. Osteomyelitis in the diabetic foot rarely occurs without a portal of entry, such as an ulcer or puncture. Nuclear imaging can be helpful in differentiating osteomyelitis from Charcot foot. A useful algorithm for differentiation is shown in Figure 9.2.[17] This flowchart requires the use of imaging combined with clinical factors to produce the most accurate diagnosis. Magnetic resonance imaging is touted as highly sensitive and specific for Charcot foot and osteomyelitis. The complicating factor is that MRI is not effective at differentiating between the two conditions. Often, "secondary signs" must be present on an MRI for differential diagnosis.[18] Positron emission tomography (PET) scans are being investigated as a modality that can be used as a single test to differentiate Charcot joint disease from osteomyelitis.[19]

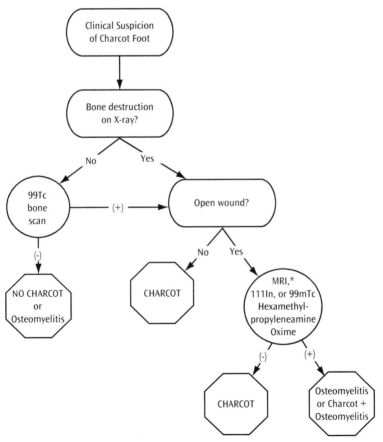

Figure 9.2—A flowchart for the radiographic investigation of the Charcot joint and differentiation from osteomyelitis. Reproduced with permission from Rogers and Bevilacqua.[20]

Classification of the Charcot Foot

The most commonly referenced classification of Charcot's arthropathy is based on radiographic findings associated with stages of the disease process. The Eichenholtz classification divides the disease into three radiographically distinct stages: development, coalescence, and reconstruction.[21] The development stage represents the acute destructive phase of this disease and is characterized by soft tissue swelling, intra-articular fractures, osteochondral fragmentation, or joint dislocation. The coalescence stage represents the reparative phase of healing and is marked by a reduction in soft tissue swelling, bone callus proliferation, consolidation of bony fragments, and healing of fractures. Finally, the reconstruction stage reflects further repair and remodeling of bone and is evidenced by bony ankylosis and hypertrophic proliferation.

Eichenholtz's radiographic classification is descriptive, but it has limited clinical value. In practice, the stage of development is considered active, whereas the stages of coalescence and reconstruction are quiescent or inactive. This classification fails to identify the earliest presentation of the Charcot foot (before the development of radiographic evidence), the location involved, and the association with ulcers. However, a stage 0 classification has been proposed, corresponding to the prodromal period of the Charcot foot seen in a high-risk patient. The classification describes a locally swollen, warm, and erythematous foot with absent, minimal, or very subtle radiographic changes.[7,22] The international task force on the Charcot foot recommended using a simple clinical classification as "active" (inflamed) or "inactive."[23]

A descriptive anatomical classification of the Charcot foot based on patterns of bone and joint destruction has been described.[1,24,25] Although this approach to classification does not indicate the stage or activity of disease, it more precisely identifies anatomic sites of involvement and the association of foot deformity with plantar ulceration. Five characteristic patterns (Fig. 9.3) range from the forefoot (pattern I) to the tarsometatarsal joints (pattern II), the lesser tarsus (pattern III), the ankle and subtalar joints (pattern IV), and the posterior calcaneus (pattern V). Patterns I and II are frequently associated with deformity and ulceration. Joint involvement is most frequently seen in patterns I, II, and III, with the most severe structural deformity and functional instability associated with patterns II and IV.

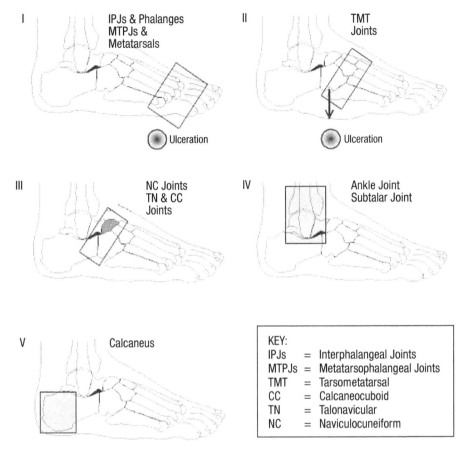

Figure 9.3—Five anatomical patterns of bone and joint involvement commonly reported in patients with diabetic neuropathic osteoarthropathy (Charcot's joint disease). Reproduced with permission from Sanders and Frykberg.[25]

Management of the Charcot Foot

Management of the Charcot foot is determined by the activity of the disease (active versus inactive), the anatomical pattern of bone and joint involvement, and the degree of involvement (such as deformity, fractures, fragmentation of bone, and instability), as well as the presence of ulceration and wound infection. Immobilization and reduction of weight-bearing stress are the foundations of treatment for acute Charcot foot.[23] Although some experts recommend non–weight-bearing on the affected extremity, several studies indicate that weight-bearing in a total contact cast is not detrimental.[26,27] Offloading the foot effectively reduces further trauma, yet this strategy may at the same time increase stress on the contralateral limb. This, in turn, may precipitate neuropathic fractures and ulceration on the previously unaffected foot. The risk of bilateral Charcot foot in individuals affected is up to 30%.

Reduced skin temperature and swelling are markers of healing. Skin temperatures can be monitored by noncontact infrared thermometry or thermal imaging. When the temperature difference between the same point on extremities is <4°F (2.5°C), protected weight-bearing is permitted, usually with a total contact cast, walking brace, or patellar tendon–bearing orthosis.[28] Patients can then ambulate safely while bony consolidation and remodeling take place. Mean treatment time (casting followed by protected weight-bearing in a removable cast walker) before the return to therapeutic footwear is approximately 4–6 months.

Other treatments under investigation include pharmacologic therapy of the Charcot foot with bisphosphonates or calcitonin to inhibit osteoclastic activity.[29,30] When the international task force on the Charcot foot met in 2010, there was consensus among the panelists that available pharmacotherapies did not have sufficient evidence to justify their recommendation in patients with Charcot foot.[23] Similarly, managing acute cases with ancillary bone stimulators to promote more rapid consolidation of fractures has been explored.[31] Although promising, these adjunctive treatments have not been conclusively proven effective through large, prospective, randomized clinical trials.

Surgical Management

Surgery should be considered when deformity or instability of the foot cannot be accommodated or controlled by prescription footwear or bracing.[23] Advances in surgical techniques and fixation have improved outcomes, but complication rates are still high.[32,33] Surgical approaches to treatment range from isolated Achilles tendon lengthening, with or without simple ostectomy, to major reconstruction of the foot with open-reduction and fixation of fractures and dislocations by internal or external means. External skeletal fixation devices (frames) to maintain a plantigrade position of the foot during healing have proven useful in fixating the reconstructed Charcot foot, since these devices are indicated for osteopenic bone (Fig. 9.4). While long-term outcomes including functional evaluations and quality of life studies comparing *surgical* treatments are needed, the evidence is mounting that surgical management may be a beneficial adjunct to care.[34] However, the known outcomes of *nonsurgical* management are far from optimal. Saltzman et al.[35] reviewed 127 Charcot feet treated by nonsurgical means and noted a 2.7% amputation rate and 49% reulceration rate over an average of 3.8 years.

Some literature exists on the outcomes of surgical reconstruction for Charcot arthropathy. Grant et al.[36] reported on 50 Charcot feet in patients with follow-up between 2 and 5 years who underwent surgical reconstruction and found that 84% had a fusion or stable pseudo-fusion and a 4% amputation rate. Pinzur[37] reviewed 147 patients with midfoot Charcot arthropathy and found that 40% required surgical intervention to achieve the desired endpoint. Many factors must be taken into consideration, including the joint(s) involved, the medical status of the patient, the rehabilitation potential, and the frequency of postop-

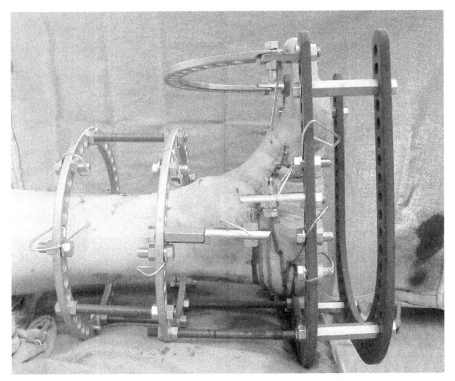

Figure 9.4—A Charcot foot status post-reconstruction with external ring fixation in place to maintain correction and compression of the arthrodesis site (midfoot).

erative complications. Bevilacqua and Rogers[38] summarized the key concepts in the surgical management of the Charcot midfoot. Ankle equinus is a common finding that compounds the severity of the joint deformity. Both the equinus and improving the lateral calcaneal inclination and talo-first metatarsal declination angles should be addressed during the surgical management.

Postoperative complications are common, occurring in nearly all patients when external fixation is used.[32,33] The complications are usually pin tract infections and wire breakage. The occurrence of complications does not affect the outcome if recognized and managed appropriately.

A clinical practice pathway summarizing the diagnostic and treatment considerations for the diabetic Charcot foot is illustrated in Fig. 9.5.[23]

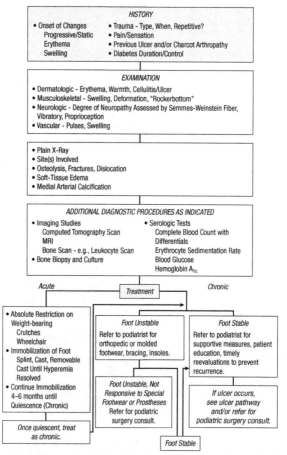

Figure 9.5—An algorithm depicting the basic approach to the treatment of the Charcot foot.[23]

Summary

Charcot's joint disease of the foot and ankle is a serious complication of diabetes that is unfortunately frequently misdiagnosed and often debilitating. Some have classified this condition as a "medical emergency," since there are therapies available that can alter its natural history.[39] Diagnosis is made based on clinical suspicion of the disorder in high-risk patients. Successful treatment hinges on early recognition, immobilization, and offloading until inflammation has subsided and the foot is stable. Therapeutic footwear and bracing are integral components of treatment. Nonsurgical management of the Charcot foot remains the most desirable approach for most patients. Surgical intervention is generally reserved for the most recalcitrant cases, including patients with instability, recurrent ulcerations, or complicating osteomyelitis.

Nevertheless, primary prevention of the Charcot foot should be our objective. Patient and physician education regarding foot inspection, risk factors, and metabolic control of diabetes, as well as pharmacotherapy for the prevention of peripheral neuropathy, may facilitate this goal.

References

1. Sanders LJ, Frykberg RG. The Charcot foot (pied de Charcot). In *Levin and O'Neal's The Diabetic Foot*. 7th ed. Bowker J, Pfeifer MA, Eds. Philadelphia, Elsevier, 2008, p. 257

2. Charcot J-M. Sur quelques arthropathies qui paraissent dépendre d'une lésion du cerveau ou de la moelle épinière. *Arch Physio Norm Pathol* 1868;1:161–178

3. Charcot J-M. Demonstration of arthropathic affections of locomotor ataxy. *BMJ* 1881;2:285

4. Page HW. Joint disease in a case of Tabes Dorsalis (Locomotor ataxy). In *Transactions of the International Medical Congress: Seventh Session Held in London, August 2–9, 1881*. Vol. 1. MacCormac W, Klockmann JW, Eds. London, U.K., Balantyne, Hanson & Company, 1881, p. 124

5. Charcot J-M, Féré C. Affections osseuses et articulaires du pied chez les tabétiques (Pied tabétique). *Archives de Neurologie* 1883;6:305–319

6. Stevens MJ, Edmonds ME, Foster AV, Watkins PJ. Selective neuropathy

and preserved vascular responses in the diabetic Charcot foot. *Diabetologia* 1992;35:148–154

7. Shibata T, Tada K, Hashizume C. The results of arthrodesis of the ankle for leprotic neuroarthropathy. *J Bone Joint Surg Am* 1990;72:749–756

8. Frykberg RG, Belczyk R. Epidemiology of the Charcot foot. *Clin Podiatr Med Surg* 2008;25:17–28

9. Lavery LA, Armstrong DG, Wunderlich RP, et al. Diabetic foot syndrome: evaluating the prevalence and incidence of foot pathology in Mexican Americans and non-Hispanic whites from a diabetes management cohort. *Diabetes Care* 2003;26:1435–1438

10. Cavanagh PR, Young MJ, Adams JE, et al. Radiographic abnormalities in the feet of patients with diabetic neuropathy. *Diabetes Care* 1994;17:201–209

11. Brower AC, Allman RM. Pathogenesis of the neurotrophic joint: neurotraumatic vs. neurovascular. *Radiology* 1981;139:349–354

12. Mabilleau G, Petrova NL, Edmonds ME, Sabokbar A. Increased osteoclastic activity in acute Charcot's osteoarthropathy: the role of receptor activator of nuclear factor-kappa B ligand. *Diabetologia* 2008; 51:1035–1040

13. Petrova NL, Moniz C, Elias DA, et al. Is there a systemic inflammatory response in the acute Charcot foot? *Diabetes Care* 2007;30:997–998

14. Pitocco D, Zelano G, Gioffrè G, et al. Association between osteoprotegerin G1181C and T245G polymorphisms and diabetic Charcot neuroarthropathy: a case-control study. *Diabetes Care* 2009;32:1694–1697

15. Pakarinen TK, Laine HJ, Honkonen SE, et al. Charcot arthropathy of the diabetic foot: current concepts and review of 36 cases. *Scand J Surg* 2002;91:195–201

16. Chantelau E. The perils of procrastination: effects of early vs. delayed detection and treatment of incipient Charcot fracture. *Diabet Med* 2005;22:1707–1712

17. Rogers LC, Bevilacqua NJ. The diagnosis of Charcot foot. *Clin Podiatr Med Surg* 2008;25:43–51

18. Morrison WB, Schweitzer ME, Batte WG, et al. Osteomyelitis of the foot: relative importance of primary and secondary MR imaging signs. *Radiology* 1998;207:625–632

19. Keidar Z, Militianu D, Melamed E, et al. The diabetic foot: initial experience with 18F-FDG PET/CT. *J Nucl Med* 2005;46:444–449

20. Rogers LC, Bevilacqua NJ. Imaging of the Charcot foot. *Clin Pod Med Surg* 2008;25:263–274

21. Eichenholtz SN. *Charcot Joints.* Springfield, IL, Charles C. Thomas, 1966

22. Sella EJ, Barrette C. Staging of Charcot neuroarthropathy along the medial column of the foot in the diabetic patient. *J Foot Ankle Surg* 1999;38:34–40

23. Rogers LC, Frykberg RG, Armstrong DG, et al. The Charcot foot in diabetes. *Diabetes Care* 2011;34:2123–2129

24. Sanders LJ, Mrdjenovich D. Anatomical patterns of bone and joint destruction in neuropathic diabetics (Abstract). *Diabetes* 40(Suppl. 1): 529A, 1991

25. Sanders LJ, Frykberg RG. Diabetic neuropathic osteoarthropathy: the Charcot foot. In *The High Risk Foot in Diabetes Mellitus.* Frykberg RG, Ed. New York, Churchill Livingstone, 1991, p. 297

26. Pinzur MS, Lio T, Posner M. Treatment of Eichenholtz stage I Charcot foot arthro-pathy with a weightbearing total contact cast. *Foot Ankle Int* 2006;27:324–329

27. de Souza LJ. Charcot arthropathy and immobilization in a weight-bearing total contact cast. *J Bone Joint Surg Am* 2008;90:754–759

28. Rogers LC, Frykberg RG. The Charcot foot. *Med Clin North Am* 2013;97:847–856

29. Jude EB, Selby PL, Burgess J, et al. Bisphosphonates in the treatment of Charcot neuroarthropathy: a double-blind randomised controlled trial. *Diabetologia* 2001;44:2032–2037

30. Bem R, Jirkovská A, Fejfarová V, et al. Intranasal calcitonin in the treatment of acute Charcot neuroosteoarthropathy: a randomized controlled trial. *Diabetes Care* 2006;29:1392–1394

31. Frykberg RG, Zgonis T, Armstrong DG, et al.; American College of Foot and Ankle Surgeons. Diabetic foot disorders: a clinical practice guideline (2006 revision). *J Foot Ankle Surg* 2006;45(Suppl. 5):S1–S66

32. Rogers LC, Bevilacqua NJ, Frykberg RG, Armstrong DG. Predictors of postoperative complications of Ilizarov external ring fixators in the foot and ankle. *J Foot Ankle Surg* 2007;46:372–375

33. Wukich DK, Belczyk RJ, Burns PR, Frykberg RG. Complications encountered with circular ring fixation in persons with diabetes mellitus. *Foot Ankle Int* 2008;29:994–1000

34. Najafi B, Crews RT, Armstrong DG, et al. Can we predict outcome of surgical reconstruction of Charcot neuroarthropathy by dynamic plantar pressure assessment? A proof of concept study. *Gait Posture.* 2010;31:87–92

35. Saltzman CL, Hagy ML, Zimmerman B, et al. How effective is intensive nonoperative initial treatment of patients with diabetes and Charcot arthropathy of the feet? *Clin Orthop Relat Res* 2005;435:185–190

36. Grant WP, Garcia-Lavin SE, Sabo RT, et al. A retrospective analysis of 50 consecutive Charcot diabetic salvage reconstructions. *J Foot Ankle Surg* 2009;48:30–38

37. Pinzur M. Surgical versus accommodative treatment for Charcot arthropathy of the midfoot. *Foot Ankle Int* 2004;25:545–549

38. Bevilacqua NJ, Rogers LC. Surgical management of Charcot midfoot deformities. *Clin Pod Med Surg* 2008;25:81–94

39. Tan AL, Greenstein A, Jarrett SJ, McGonagle D. Acute neuropathic joint disease: a medical emergency? *Diabetes Care* 2005;28:2962–2964

Suggested Readings

Hanft JR, Goggin JP, Landsman A, Surprenant M. The role of combined magnetic field bone growth stimulation as an adjunct in the treatment of neuroarthropathy/Charcot joint: an expanded pilot study. *J Foot Ankle Surg* 1998;37:510–515

Hoché G, Sanders LJ. On some arthropathies apparently related to a lesion of the brain or spinal cord, by Dr. J.-M. Charcot, January 1868. Translation of Charcot's original 1868 paper on tabetic arthropathies. *J Hist Neurosci* 1992;1:75–87

Sanders LJ. What lessons can history teach us about the Charcot foot? *Clin Podiatric Med Surg* 2008;25:1–15

10
Infection in the Diabetic Foot

Edgar J.G. Peters, MD, PhD,[1] and Benjamin A. Lipsky, MD, FACP, FIDSA, FRCP[2]
[1]Department of Medicine, Section of Infectious Diseases, University of Amsterdam, the Netherlands; and [2]University of Washington, Seattle, WA

Foot infections in individuals with diabetes cause substantial financial cost, morbidity, and reduced quality of life and are the most common event leading to lower-limb amputation.[1] Infection generally begins in a foot wound, most often a neuropathic and/or ischemic ulceration, emphasizing the importance of prevention and treatment of foot ulcers.[2] Foot infections must be addressed promptly and effectively, since delay increases the risk of spreading to deeper soft tissues, bone involvement, and a resultant poor outcome.[3,4] Uncertainties persist on many issues, but several international committees have produced consensus guidelines that offer a framework for assessing and treating diabetic foot soft tissue and bone infections.[3–5]

Epidemiology

Foot ulceration is the major risk factor for infection, but in only 40–80% of cases are they clinically infected at presentation.[1,6] Peripheral neuropathy, peripheral arterial disease, and perhaps other comorbidities, such as suboptimal glycemic control, appear to increase the risk of infection.[7] Approximately one-fifth of infections involve bone (osteomyelitis), and about one-third are classified as severe (see below) at presentation. Infection is now the main reason for diabetes-related hospitalization and is the usual immediate precipitating factor for nontraumatic lower-extremity amputations.[8]

DOI: 10.2337/9781580405706.10

Definitions

Understanding the relationship between pathogenic bacteria and the human host is essential in formulating infection management strategies.[9,10]

- **Contamination** of a wound occurs when potentially pathogenic bacteria are introduced into exposed host tissue. Any type of trauma that disrupts the protective skin envelope can lead to contamination. The number and virulence of the organisms and the robustness of the host's immune system determine the outcome of this event.
- **Colonization** occurs when bacteria in an ulcer replicate and establish a physiological state of coexistence without overt tissue damage or host response.
- **Infection** is diagnosed when contaminating or colonizing microorganisms invade host tissue, inciting an inflammatory response and causing cellular and tissue damage.
- **Diabetic foot infection** refers to infection involving the skin, soft tissue, bones, or joints below the malleoli in a person with diabetes.

Diagnosis

Because bacteria can be isolated from both contaminated/colonized wounds and infected tissues, clinical criteria are usually used to diagnose infection. The results of microbiological tests (i.e., cultures or molecular techniques) can only be used diagnostically when specimens are taken from sites that have no resident flora (i.e., deep, viable tissues) by methods that minimize sampling of colonized areas and that avoid contamination during sampling. Microbiology is, of course, crucial to identify the causative pathogens and their antibiotic susceptibilities in clinically infected wounds.

The clinical diagnosis of infection requires evidence of the host sustaining tissue damage and initiating an inflammatory response. Consensus criteria for diagnosing infection of a diabetic foot wound are the presence of two or more of the following findings[5]:

- Local swelling or induration
- Erythema (>0.5 cm from the ulcer margin)
- Local tenderness or pain
- Local warmth
- Purulent discharge (pus)

The presence of peripheral neuropathy or vasculopathy can, unfortunately, obscure or mimic the signs and symptoms of inflammation. Thus, some define infection by the presence of colonization with high numbers of organisms (typically $\geq 10^5$ colony-forming units/gram tissue) or evidence of other possible "secondary" signs of infection, including a wound that fails to heal as expected despite appropriate treatment; excessive or abnormal ulcer drainage; friable, discolored, or pocketed granulation tissue; an abnormally foul smell; the development of wound necrosis; or high concentrations of bacteria on the wound surface.[10,11]

Clinical Manifestations and Classification

Types of infection range from paronychia (an inflammation around an ingrown toenail) to infections of ulcers, deep soft tissue compartments, fascial planes, tendon sheaths, joints, and bones. Because anatomic schemes are inadequate to establish priorities for clinical management, two consensus groups developed a now-validated scheme that classifies infections according to their severity[4,5,8]:

- **Uninfected** ulcers do not meet the criteria outlined above for the clinical diagnosis of infection. While they need treatment, they usually pose no immediate threat to limb or patient and do not require antimicrobial therapy.
- **Mild infections** involve only the skin and superficial subcutaneous tissue. Any erythema extends <2 cm from the ulcer margin, and any necrosis is minimal. These infections should be cultured and treated (including with antimicrobials), but pose minimal immediate risk.
- **Moderate infections** are a heterogeneous group. They include individuals in which erythema extends >2 cm beyond the ulcer border or in which infection breaches the superficial fascia and hence involves deeper structures, including tendon, bone, or joint. There may be deep abscesses, necrosis, or gangrene but the patient lacks criteria for the systemic inflammatory response syndrome. These infections often pose immediate risk to the foot and require urgent treatment.
- **Severe infections** are clinically similar to moderate ones in anatomic extent, but the patient manifests a systemic inflammatory response in the form of fever, leukocytosis, tachycardia, tachypnea, hypotension, or marked metabolic derangements. Because these responses are often muted in

people with longstanding diabetes, their presence suggests more serious disease, potentially including bacteremia. In addition to being limb-threatening, severe infections can pose immediate threat to life.

This classification scheme, by the Infectious Diseases Society of America guideline committee, correspond directly to grades 1 (uninfected) to 4 (severe) of the diabetic foot ulcer classification scheme produced for research purposes by the International Working Group on the Diabetic Foot.[5,12] To categorize the case mix of ulcers studied in trials, this latter scheme considers perfusion, extent of ulcer (area), depth of the wound, presence of infection (graded for severity as noted above), and sensation, which together make the acronym PEDIS. The presence of clinically significant limb ischemia increases the threat posed by any stage of infection.

Assessment

Optimal treatment of the infection requires carefully considering not only the foot, but also the leg and person to whom it is (and, hopefully, will remain) attached. The clinician must assess the following:

- *The patient:* Vital signs; cognitive function; psychosocial situation; understanding of, and engagement with, his or her own health care needs; availability of other caregivers
- *The limb:* Arterial perfusion, extent and rapidity of any proximal spread of infection
- *The foot:* Biomechanics, neuropathy, ischemia, evidence of deep space infections or extensive soft tissue involvement, bony deformity
- *The wound:* Extent, depth, presence of necrosis, involvement of bone, joint, or tendon

Assessing the wound may require some debridement of callus, ulcer slough, and necrotic tissue (eschar). If a sterile blunt metal probe introduced into the ulcer strikes rock-hard, gritty material (a positive "probe to bone" test), there is a moderate likelihood of osteomyelitis when clinical suspicion is high, whereas a negative test in a patient at low risk makes osteomyelitis unlikely.[13] Probing the wound can also reveal loose bony fragments, foreign bodies, and communications into joints or deep spaces. Plain X-rays of the foot are useful for evaluating for bony involvement, soft tissue gas, and foreign bodies in most infected lesions. They are often adequate for imaging, but if the patient could have other bony disorders (such as neuroosteoarthropathy [Charcot foot]) or if it is important to know the extent of the soft tissue infection, magnetic resonance imaging (MRI) is currently the best of the available diagnostic imaging studies.[14,15] Newer imaging methods (such as SPECT/CT, PET) are promising, but their relative merits have not been adequately investigated.[14,16] Obtaining blood for a complete blood count and tests of inflammatory markers (erythrocyte sedimentation rate, C-reactive protein) may help assess the severity of the infection. For most moderate, and virtually all severe, infections, an experienced surgeon should assess the patient to determine whether any operative intervention is needed.

Microbiological Diagnosis

Because uninfected ulcers do not require antimicrobial therapy, these need not be cultured. Some acute and antibiotic-naive mild infections do not require microbiological sampling, since the pathogens are almost always aerobic grampositive cocci—typically, *Staphylococcus aureus* or beta-hemolytic streptococci.[17] However, specimens must be cultured when the infection is extensive, empiric treatment is failing, or antibiotic resistance (e.g., methicillin-resistant *S. aureus* or extended-spectrum β-lactamases) is a concern. Diabetic foot infections are often polymicrobial, including gram-negative and obligate anaerobic organisms. Obtaining specimens by aspiration of pus, curettage of tissue from the debrided ulcer base (not of slough), or biopsy of deeper tissue, rather than wound swabs, provides more accurate results. Clearly identifying the type of specimen and any antibiotic therapy the patient is currently taking or has recently taken, and rapidly transporting the specimen to the laboratory, will optimize processing and analysis of the samples. Newer molecular microbiological techniques have demonstrated that there are more bacterial species in foot wounds than standard cultures reveal, but the clinical importance of this information is as yet unclear.[18]

Treatment Planning

After assessing the severity of the infection and its key accompanying features, and considering the likely etiologic pathogens, the clinician is ready to formulate a treatment plan.[5] Most wounds need at least some debriding of necrotic tissue and surrounding callus. Surgery may be needed to drain any abscesses, or to remove more extensive areas of necrotic tissue. Wounds subjected to biomechanical plantar pressure need to be offloaded. Severe ischemia, if present, must be addressed. Metabolic disturbances, such as electrolyte imbalance or hyperglycemia, should be corrected. Many diabetic foot infections have organisms in a biofilm state, i.e., a structured community of microorganisms within an adherent, self-developed polymeric matrix, which impairs eradication with antibiotics or by the host immune system.[10] As a consequence, common practice consists of mechanical removal of these bacteria with surgical debridement. Efforts to find solutions for removal of bacteria in the biofilm phenotypic state with chemicals or local antiseptics are still under development.

The following approach should help the clinician choose the venue for patient care (ambulatory versus hospital) and an appropriate empiric antibiotic regimen[5]:

- *Uninfected ulcers* do not require antibiotic therapy, because it has not been shown to either improve ulcer healing or to prevent active infection.[19]
- *Mild infections* can be treated on an ambulatory basis, unless the patient has cognitive or social impairments affecting his or her ability to care for the ulcer and properly take antibiotic therapy. Semisynthetic penicillins (dicloxacillin, cloxacillin, flucloxacillin) or first-generation cephalosporins (e.g., cephalexin) are usually adequate for first-line treatment, unless the risk of methicillin-resistant *S. aureus* is high, in which case agents such as linezolid, trimethoprim-sulfamethoxazole, or doxycycline may be appropriate.
- *Moderate infections* needing urgent antibiotic therapy require relatively broad-spectrum empiric coverage that will be active against gram-positive cocci, as well as aerobic gram-negative rods and anaerobes. The latter organisms are more frequent in chronic and complex infections, which have often failed to respond to prior antibiotic therapy. Appropriate choices include combinations of a fluoroquinolone (e.g., ciprofloxacin, levofloxacin, or moxifloxacin) with clindamycin or a penicillin/penicillinase inhibitor (e.g., ampicillin-sulbactam or amoxicillin-clavulanate). Because susceptibility to antimicrobial drugs varies among geographical areas and patient populations, the choice of empiric antibiotic therapy should consider local patterns.[20] Only select patients (e.g., those with previous antibiotic therapy, who live in hot climates, or who have extensive

water-related exposure) need empiric coverage for *Pseudomonas aeruginosa*. Hospitalization may be required for a surgical procedure or, occasionally, for special diagnostic tests. For chronic, stable infections (e.g., osteomyelitis), it is often better to withhold antibiotic therapy until proper cultures can be obtained and processed.

- *Severe infections* must always be treated urgently, with hospitalization and initial intravenous antibiotics. The selected antimicrobial regimen should cover the above-cited organisms as well as *Pseudomonas aeruginosa* and potentially other resistant aerobic gram-negative rods. Appropriate regimens include a carbapenem (e.g., imipenem-cilastatin or meropenem) or antipseudomonal penicillins with a β-lactamase inhibitor (e.g., piperacillin-tazobactam). Always consider the potential need for surgery in addition to the medical treatment and to treat any metabolic or other systemic effects of infection.

Adjunctive treatments (e.g., hyperbaric oxygen, granulocyte-colony stimulating factors, and negative-pressure wound therapy) have not been shown to improve outcomes of infection, but may be considered in appropriately selected patients.[21]

Osteomyelitis

Diagnosing and treating osteomyelitis are particularly difficult tasks.[5,22] Bony abnormalities may not be seen on plain X-rays in the first few weeks of bone infection.[14] On the other hand, noninfectious neuropathic (Charcot) osteoarthropathy, which causes radiographic changes that can mimic infection, is frequently present in individuals with longstanding diabetes. Most radionuclide isotope scans are insufficiently sensitive and specific to distinguish between the two conditions, although modern forms of white-cell labeling show promise.[23] Magnetic resonance imaging currently offers the most accurate diagnosis when properly interpreted.[14,15] Promising imaging tests include positron emission tomography/computed tomography and SPECT/CT scans, but there have been relatively few studies of these modalities to date.[14,16]

Treatment of osteomyelitis traditionally requires both surgical resection of infected or necrotic bone and prolonged antibiotic therapy. The advent of highly bioavailable oral antibiotics has substantially reduced, if not eliminated, the required duration of intravenous therapy. In several retrospective reviews, and some prospective (including one randomized controlled) trials, diabetic foot osteomyelitis was arrested by antibiotic therapy without concomitant surgery in 60–70% of patients.[24-26] In each case, clinicians, in collaboration with their patients, must decide whether predominantly antibiotic, versus surgical, therapy is most appropriate.

Duration of Therapy

The severity of infection and the presence of bony involvement largely determine the recommended length of treatment. Antibiotic therapy is indicated for treating infection, not for healing a wound, which takes much longer. If the infection does not respond as expected, reassess the patient's adherence to the antibiotic and ulcer care regimens and check for any undetected abscess, necrosis, or ischemia. Recommended durations of therapy are as follows[5]:

- **Mild soft tissue infections:** usually 1–2 weeks, usually entirely oral
- **Moderate soft tissue infections:** typically 1–3 weeks (if no bone involvement), often with initial short-term parenteral, followed by a switch to oral, therapy
- **Severe soft tissue infections:** 1–3 weeks, always initially parenteral, depending on the nature of any surgery and the presence of bacteremia
- **Osteomyelitis:** Duration depends on the extent of residual bone involvement after any surgical intervention:
  - All involved bone is removed (ablative surgery): treatment based on any soft tissue involvement; if uninfected, prophylaxis for up to 72 h; if infected, treat for 2 weeks
  - Infected but viable bone remains: 4–6 weeks
  - Dead bone remains: minimum of 6–12 weeks. Long-term antibiotic regimens are sometimes used to suppress, rather than attempt to cure, infection

Summary

To help avoid encouraging antibiotic resistance, the length and breadth of antibiotic therapy should be tailored to the severity of the infection; choose the narrowest spectrum and shortest duration appropriate. If treatment fails or progress is slow, reevaluate the wound as well as the patient, rather than reflexively adding additional agents. Future studies need to establish the most cost-effective diagnostic and treatment strategies, especially in relation to osteomyelitis.

References

1. Prompers L, Huijberts M, Apelqvist J, et al. High prevalence of isch-aemia, infection and serious comorbidity in patients with diabetic foot disease in Europe: baseline results from the Eurodiale study. *Diabetologia* 2007;50:18–25

2. Boulton AJ, Kirsner RS, Vileikyte L. Clinical practice: neuropathic dia-betic foot ulcers. *N Engl J Med* 2004;351:48–55

3. Tan T, Shaw EJ, Siddiqui F, et al. Inpatient management of diabetic foot problems: summary of NICE guidance. *BMJ* 2011;342:d1280

4. Lipsky BA, Peters EJ, Senneville E, et al. Expert opinion on the man-agement of infections in the diabetic foot. *Diabetes Metab Res Rev* 2012;28(Suppl. 1):163–178

5. Lipsky BA, Berendt AR, Cornia PB, et al. 2012 Infectious Diseases Soci-ety of America clinical practice guideline for the diagnosis and treatment of diabetic foot infections. *Clin Infect Dis* 2012;54:e132–e173

6. Apelqvist J. The foot in perspective. *Diabetes Metab Res* 2008;24 (Suppl. 1):S110–S115

7. Peters EJ, Lavery LA, Armstrong DG. Diabetic lower extremity infection: influence of physical, psychological, and social factors. *J Diabetes Compli-cations* 2005;19:107–112

8. Lavery LA, Armstrong DG, Murdoch DP, Peters EJ, Lipsky BA. Valida-tion of the Infectious Diseases Society of America's diabetic foot infection classification system. *Clin Infect Dis* 2007;44:562–565

9. Berendt LB. Principles and practice of antibiotic therapy of diabetic foot infections. *Diabetes Metab Res* 2000;16:S42–S46

10. Gottrup F, Apelqvist J, Bjansholt T, et al. EWMA document: antimicrobi-als and non-healing wounds: evidence, controversies and suggestions. *J Wound Care* 2013;22:S1–S89

11. Gardner SE, Frantz RA. Wound bioburden and infection-related compli-cations in diabetic foot ulcers. *Biol Res Nurs* 2008;10:44–53

12. Schaper NC. Diabetic foot ulcer classification system for research purposes:

a progress report on criteria for including patients in research studies. *Diabetes Metab Res* 2004;20(Suppl. 1):90–95

13. Lavery LA, Armstrong DG, Peters EJ, Lipsky BA. Probe-to-bone test for diagnosing diabetic foot osteomyelitis: reliable or relic? *Diabetes Care* 2007;30:270–274

14. Dinh MT, Abad CL, Safdar N. Diagnostic accuracy of the physical examination and imaging tests for osteomyelitis underlying diabetic foot ulcers: meta-analysis. *Clin Infect Dis* 2008;47:519–527

15. Kapoor A, Page S, Lavalley M, et al. Magnetic resonance imaging for diagnosing foot osteomyelitis: a meta-analysis. *Arch Intern Med* 2007;167:125–132

16. Capriotti G, Chianelli M, Signore A. Nuclear medicine imaging of diabetic foot infection: results of meta-analysis. *Nucl Med Commun* 2006;27:757–764

17. Lipsky BA. Empirical therapy for diabetic foot infections: are there clinical clues to guide antibiotic selection? *Clin Microbiol Infect* 2007;13:351–353

18. Lipsky BA, Richard JL, Lavigne JP. Diabetic foot ulcer microbiome: one small step for molecular microbiology: one giant leap for understanding diabetic foot ulcers? *Diabetes* 2013;62:679–681

19. Berendt AR, Lipsky BA. Should antibiotics be used in the treatment of the diabetic foot? *Diabetic Foot* 2003;6:18–28

20. de Vries MG, Ekkelenkamp MB, Peters EJ. Are clindamycin and ciprofloxacin appropriate for the empirical treatment of diabetic foot infections? *Eur J Clin Microbiol Infect Dis* 2014;33:453–456

21. Peters EJ, Lipsky BA, Berendt AR, et al. A systematic review of the effectiveness of interventions in the management of infection in the diabetic foot. *Diabetes Metab Res Rev* 2012;28(Suppl. 1):142–162

22. Berendt AR, Peters EJ, Bakker K, et al. Diabetic foot osteomyelitis: a progress report on diagnosis and a systematic review of treatment. *Diabetes Metab Res Rev* 2008;24(Suppl. 1);S145–S161

23. Palestro CJ, Love C. Nuclear medicine and diabetic foot infections. *Semin Nucl Med* 2009;39:52–65

24. Embil JM, Rose G, Trepman E, et al. Oral antimicrobial therapy for diabetic foot osteomyelitis. *Foot Ankle International* 2006;27;771–779

25. Lazaro-Martinez JL, Aragon-Sanchez J, Garcia-Morales E. Antibiotics versus conservative surgery for treating diabetic foot osteomyelitis: a randomized comparative trial. *Diabetes Care* 2014;37:789–795

26. Game FL, Jeffcoate WJ. Primarily non-surgical management of osteomyelitis of the foot in diabetes. *Diabetologia* 2008;51:962–967

11
Evaluation and Management of Peripheral Artery Disease

Joseph L. Mills, Sr., MD
Michael E. DeBakey Department of Surgery, Division of Vascular and Endovascular Surgery, Baylor College of Medicine, Houston, TX

For the almost 29 million individuals with diabetes in the United States, foot problems—ulceration, infection, and ischemia—are major causes of hospitalization. Most of these problems are a result of neuropathy, repetitive trauma, and superimposed infection. Although the classic teaching has long been that the underlying pathophysiology of diabetic foot ulcer (DFU) is related to neuropathy and loss of protective sensation (i.e., neuropathic), it has become evident that in modern practice, at least in the western world, the majority of DFUs are neuroischemic. Detectable peripheral artery disease potentially contributes to wound formation or failure to heal in nearly 50–75% of cases.[1,2] In 2007, the total direct annual health care cost of diabetes in the United States was a staggering $116 billion; approximately 20% of these expenditures were related specifically to the treatment of diabetic foot problems.[3,4]

Arteriosclerosis Obliterans

Serial clinical studies have noted the development of arteriosclerosis obliterans (ASO) in 50% of patients with type 2 diabetes within 15 years of disease onset.[5] The prevalence of ASO is 12–28 times greater than that observed in age- and sex-matched control groups.[4] Additional risk factors that are associated not only with increased prevalence but also with progression of ASO in patients with type 2 diabetes include cigarette smoking, diabetes duration >10 years,

DOI: 10.2337/9781580405706.11

HDL cholesterol <40 mg/dL, systolic blood pressure >145 mmHg, and obesity index >2.83 g/cm.[3,6,7]

Myths about ASO

Several myths about peripheral arterial disease in diabetic patients remain pervasive in the medical and patient communities and have been difficult to dispel. ASO in patients with diabetes is histologically indistinguishable from that of individuals without diabetes.[7] The major and clinically important difference is disease distribution. In individuals without diabetes, proximal arterial occlusive disease (aorto-iliac segments and distal superficial femoral artery) is more common, whereas in diabetic patients, ASO commonly affects the deep femoral artery and the medium-sized, below-knee popliteal and tibio-peroneal arteries (infrageniculate vessels).

Diabetic patients commonly present with foot ulcers or gangrene, palpable femoral and popliteal pulses, and absent foot pulses; the cause, however, is not microvascular disease, but rather ASO in the infrageniculate, or "trifurcation," vessels. The distal peroneal, dorsal pedal, and digital arteries are frequently spared, and the peroneal and pedal vessels are often sites for bypass graft insertion.

There remains a widespread misconception that patients with diabetes have arteriolar occlusive disease that can cause pedal ischemia and gangrene, even in the presence of palpable pedal pulses. The myth of a unique "diabetic microangiopathy" stems from a single amputation study reported in 1959 that demonstrated periodic acid–Schiff (PAS)-positive material in the arterioles of diabetic patients who had undergone major limb amputation.[8] Subsequent detailed angiographic, physiologic, and histological studies have not confirmed the presence of a unique diabetic microangiopathy.[3,9,10]

Although studies have confirmed that patients with diabetes have an abnormally thickened capillary basement membrane, this membrane does not appear to be associated with gangrene.[3] In fact, despite this abnormality, the patency and limb salvage results of lower-extremity bypass in patients with diabetes are equivalent to results in patients without diabetes,[11] with the exception of individuals with end-stage renal disease.[12] This observation argues strongly against the presence of clinically significant "small-vessel disease," or microangiopathy.

Treating Infection

Management of neuropathy (offloading, callus debridement, and proper footwear) and infection (appropriate antibiotics and surgical debridement) is discussed elsewhere in this book and is critical to preventing major limb amputation. Infection should be promptly and aggressively treated; wide, open debridements are frequently needed to drain purulence and remove necrotic tissue. Assessing the vascularity of every patient presenting with foot ulceration, infection, or frank gangrene and promptly recognizing and quantifying ischemia are essential. Repeated debridement of a nonhealing ischemic foot is a clinically unacceptable practice destined to result in major limb amputation.

Pulse Palpation and Noninvasive Vascular Testing

The most important component of the physical examination, from a vascular surgeon's standpoint, is peripheral pulse palpation. The presence of clearly palpable dorsal pedal and posterior tibial pulses usually indicates adequate circulation. Sufficient debridement and control of infection heal 90% of cases.

All patients lacking palpable foot pulses should undergo noninvasive testing such as Doppler-derived ankle pressure measurement and ankle-brachial index determination, digital or toe pressure measurements, pulse volume recordings, or transcutaneous oxygen measurements ($TcPo_2$). Unfortunately, because of extensive medial calcification, pedal pulses may not be palpable in some individuals with diabetes (10–20%), and ankle-pressure measurements may also be unreliable if the calcification is sufficiently severe to preclude arterial compression by the cuff (resulting in falsely elevated or suprasystolic pressures). Because the digital arteries are often spared, digital waveform and pressure measurements can be useful—we routinely perform them on all patients with foot problems and diabetes. Pulse volume recordings are helpful because they are unaffected by the presence of arterial wall calcification. Diabetic patients with an absolute ankle pressure <90 mmHg and toe pressures <55 mmHg are unlikely to heal without revascularization.[11]

Although the perfusion required for healing a foot ulcer depends on a multitude of factors (e.g., size and location of ulcer, presence and extent of gangrene and/or infection, and patient nutritional status), in general, the likelihood of healing based on objective tests of arterial perfusion follows an S-shaped curve (Fig. 11.1). At extremely low levels of perfusion (bottom left portion of curve), healing is unlikely without revascularization. If perfusion is near normal (top right portion of curve), vascular supply is adequate and healing can be reliably predicted if infection is controlled and proper wound care and offloading are performed. Foot perfusion in many patients, however, lies on the steep central portion of the sigmoid perfusion curve. In these cases, careful coordination of care with a vascular surgeon is critical to determine whether wound care alone will suffice or revascularization is necessary to ensure or expedite healing. The selection of appropriate revascularization procedure, particularly with regard to open bypass versus endoluminal therapy, or whether single level or more complete multilevel revascularization will be required, depends on an estimate of how far up the perfusion curve the foot needs to be pushed to achieve healing. Shallow nonhealing, but uninfected, forefoot ulcers may only need a small improvement in perfusion to heal, whereas multilevel revascularization or pedal bypass may be the most appropriate option for patients with extensive tissue necrosis. The concept of "critical limb ischemia" was never intended to be applied to patients with diabetes and has led to inappropriate or delayed therapy in many patients.[13,14] In recognition of this issue, the Society for Vascular Surgery (SVS) recently reclassified lower-extremity ischemia in relationship to wounds, particularly in the rapidly increasing popu-

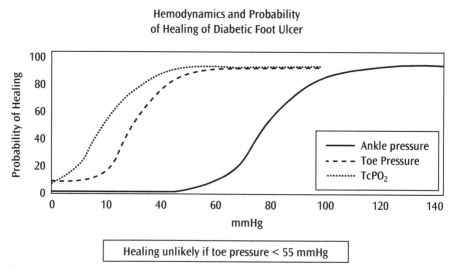

Figure 11.1—Probability of healing of a diabetic foot ulcer based on noninvasive vascular testing.

lation of patients with diabetes. The SVS lower-extremity threatened limb classification system is based on three components: wound (W), ischemia (I), and foot infection (FI) and has been termed WIFI. The ability of this new system to predict amputation risk and need for revascularization was independently validated in three reports.[15-17] The principal concepts of this system should be broadly applied in clinical practice.

Surgical and Endovascular Revascularization Options

Patients without foot pulses, with abnormal noninvasive studies, or who fail to heal despite having a foot pulse should be referred to a vascular surgeon. Subsets of patients may have hemodynamically significant tibial artery occlusive disease, despite the presence of a foot pulse, and other individuals, particularly those with end-stage renal disease and heel ulcers, may have regional ischemia of the forefoot or hindfoot[18] that can be corrected by angioplasty, if focal, or by bypass, if more diffuse.

If noninvasive tests indicate ischemia, or if healing fails despite proper drainage and debridement, arteriography should be performed by an experienced endovascular surgeon or vascular specialist. Detailed views of the infragenicalate circulation and magnified views of the foot in at least two projections, especially the lateral one, are essential. Because the peroneal, dorsal pedal, and plantar arteries are usually spared, they are most likely to serve as the recipient artery for a bypass (Figs. 11.2 and 11.3). In limb salvage situations, bypass to the infrageniculate popliteal artery, the tibial arteries, or a pedal or plantar artery is more likely to be necessary in diabetic individuals.[19-22] Except for the insertion site dictated by the more distal distribution pattern of occlusive disease, the revascularization procedure does not differ significantly from that performed in individuals without diabetes.

If detailed angiography is performed, >97% of patients threatened with loss of limb who have not previously undergone lower-extremity bypass will be found to have reconstructible arterial disease. In nearly every case, autogenous vein grafts—preferably using the long saphenous, or even the short saphenous, or arm, veins—should be used. Vein graft patency in individuals with diabetes is equivalent to that of patients without diabetes. The myth of poor results after bypass for patients with diabetes is untrue. In fact, some experienced surgeons report that patency rates for lower-extremity bypass in patients with diabetes exceed those of patients without the condition.[11,21] In appropriately

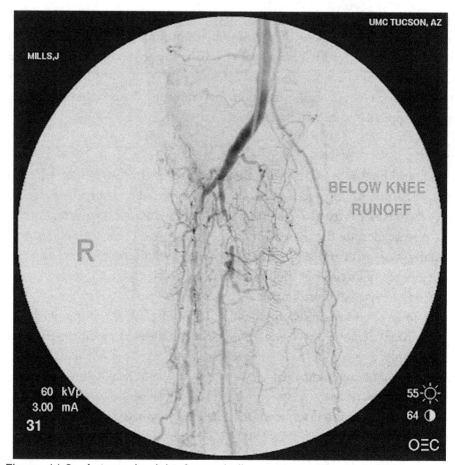

Figure 11.2—Antegrade right femoral diagnostic arteriogram (view at knee level) of an 80-year-old diabetic man with third toe gangrene, a palpable popliteal pulse, absent foot pulses, suprasystolic ankle pressures, and a great toe systolic pressure of 20 mmHg. The popliteal trifurcation is occluded, a common finding in patients with diabetes.

selected patients, revascularization is increasingly performed by endovascular means, an option that is possible in most patients, but still suffers from limited durability for tibial and long segment occlusive disease.[23] By using either open bypass or advanced endovascular techniques, most patients requiring revascularization can be helped (Fig. 11.4).

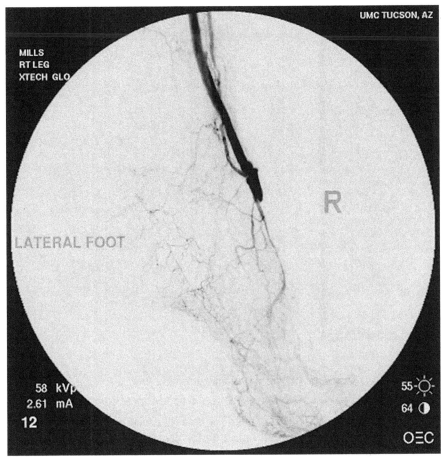

Figure 11.3—Completion arteriogram of the same patient after reversed vein bypass to the dorsalis pedis artery. Despite occlusive disease in the distal dorsalis pedis artery, the toe amputation healed (great toe pressure improved to 65 mmHg after the bypass), and the graft has remained patent for >4 years. The patient wears protective footwear and has had no recurrent foot lesions.

Summary

Patients with diabetes are 20 times more likely to have lower-extremity ASO than individuals without diabetes and are 60 times more likely to develop lower-extremity gangrene.[3] One-half to two-thirds of major limb amputations in the

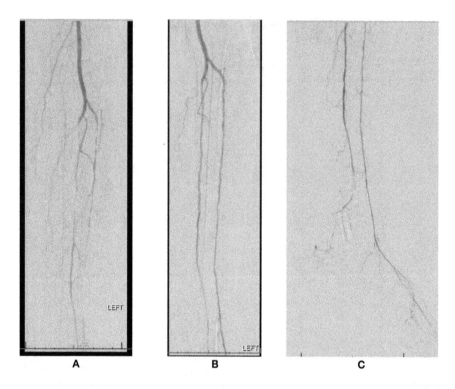

Figure 11.4—Diagnostic (A) and post-angioplasty images (B, C) of diffuse, long-segment three-vessel left trifurcation disease in a 64-year-old diabetic woman with absent pedal pulses and a forefoot wound after infection had been drained. Both the peroneal and anterior tibial arteries were successfully recanalized with 2.5 mm percutaneous balloon angioplasty.

United States are performed on patients with diabetes. Many of these amputations are the direct result of the following persistent, unfounded myths and commonly held misconceptions: *1*) gangrene results from microvascular disease, *2*) foot incisions do not heal in patients with diabetes, and *3*) bypasses do not work as well in patients with diabetes.

Abundant clinical data over the last decades suggest that none of these myths is true. Clinically important lower-extremity ischemia in patients with diabetes is caused by arteriosclerosis, and the disease pattern can usually be corrected by revascularization. Diabetic patients with foot lesions and diminished or absent foot pulses, or individuals who fail to heal despite apparently adequate circulation, should promptly be referred to an experienced vascular surgeon. Noninvasive testing and liberal use of arteriography allows significant vascular lesions to be identified and corrected. Endovascular approaches are increasingly applicable, and such techniques should be viewed as complementary to open bypass.[23] A surgical option for revascularization is available in nearly every case. Revascularization results in 75–80% limb salvage at 5 years.[19,24] Early referral and aggressive revascularization are likely to reduce substantially the number of unnecessary major limb amputations.[25]

References

1. American Diabetes Association. Peripheral arterial disease in people with diabetes (Position Statement). *Diabetes Care* 2003;26:3333–3341

2. Ndip A, Jude EB. Emerging evidence for neuroischemic diabetic foot ulcers: model of care and how to adapt practice. *Int J Low Ext Wounds* 2009;8:82–94

3. Kalish JA, Pomposelli FB. Diabetic foot problems. In *Comprehensive Vascular and Endovascular Surgery.* 2nd ed. Hallett JW, Mills JL, Earnshaw JJ, Reekers JA, Eds. New York, Elsevier, 2009, p. 215–228

4. Rogers LC, Lavery LA, Armstrong DG. The right to bear legs: an amendment to healthcare: how preventing amputations can save billions for the US Health-care System. *J Am Podiatr Med Assoc* 2008;98:166–168

5. Strandness DE. Diabetes mellitus and vascular surgery. In *Basic Data Underlying Clinical Decision Making in Vascular Surgery.* Porter JM, Taylor LM, Eds. St. Louis, MO, Quality Medical Publishing, 1994, p. 30–33

6. Beach KW, Brunzell JD, Conquest LL, Strandness DE. The correlation of arteriosclerosis obliterans with lipoproteins in insulin-dependent and non-insulin-dependent diabetes. *Diabetes* 1979;28:836–840

7. Beach KW, Strandness DE Jr. Arteriosclerosis obliterans and associated risk factors in insulin-dependent and non-insulin-dependent diabetes. *Diabetes* 1980;29:882–888

8. Beach KW, Bedford GR, Bergelin RO, et al. Progression of lower-extremity arterial occlusive disease in type II diabetes mellitus. *Diabetes Care* 1988;11:464–472

9. Strandness DE, Priest RE, Gibbons GE. Combined clinical and pathologic study of diabetic and nondiabetic peripheral arterial disease. *Diabetes* 1964;13:366–372

10. LoGerfo FW, Coffman JD. Vascular and microvascular disease of the foot in diabetes. *N Engl J Med* 1984;311:1615–1618

11. Akbari CM, Pomposelli FB Jr, Gibbons GW, et al. Lower extremity revascularization in diabetes: late observations. *Arch Surg* 2000;135:452–456

12. Johnson BL, Glickman MH, Bandyk DF, Esses GE. Failure of foot salvage in patients with end-stage renal disease after surgical revascularization. *J Vasc Surg* 1995;22:280–285, discussion 285–286

13. Bell PRF, Charlesworth D, DePalma RG, et al. The definition of critical ischaemia of a limb. Working Party of the International Vascular Symposium. *Br J Surg* 1982;69(Suppl.):S2.

14. Mills JL, Conte MS, Armstrong DG, et al. The Society for Vascular Surgery Lower Extremity Threatened Limb Classification System: risk stratification based on Wound, Ischemia and foot Infection (WIfI). *J Vasc Surg* 2014:59;220–234

15. Cull DL, Manos G, Hartley MC, et al. An early validation of the Society for Vascular Surgery Lower Extremity Threatened Limb Classification System. *J Vasc Surg* 2014;60:1535–1542

16. Causey MW, Wu B, Dini M, et al. Society for Vascular Surgery (SVS) lower extremity threatened limb classification discriminates early outcomes in hospitalized patients. *J Vasc Surg* 2014;59(6 Suppl.):103S–104S

17. Zhan LX, Branco BC, Armstrong DG, Mills JL. The Society for Vascular Surgery (SVS) lower extremity threatened limb classification system based on Wound, Ischemia, and foot Infection (WIfI) correlates with risk of major amputation and time to wound healing. *J Vasc Surg* 2015;61:939–944

18. Gentile AT, Berman SS, Reinke KR, et al. A regional pedal ischemia scoring system for decision analysis in patients with heel ulceration. *Am J Surg* 1998;176:109–114

19. Taylor LM Jr, Porter JM. Results of lower extremity bypass in the diabetic patient. *Sem Vasc Surg* 1992;5:226–233

20. Mills JL, Gahtan V, Fujitani R, et al. The utility and durability of vein bypass grafts originating from the popliteal artery for limb salvage. *Am J Surg* 1994;168:646–651

21. Pomposelli FB Jr, Jepsen SJ, Gibbons GW, et al. Efficacy of the dorsal pedal bypass for limb salvage in diabetic patients: short term observations. *J Vasc Surg* 1990;11:745–751

22. Tannenbaum GA, Pomposelli FB Jr, Marcaccio EJ, et al. Safety of vein bypass grafting to the dorsal pedal artery in diabetic patients with foot infections. *J Vasc Surg* 1992;15:982–990

23. Mills JL. Open bypass and endoluminal therapy: complementary techniques for revascularization in diabetic patients with critical limb ischemia. *Diabetes Metab Res Rev* 2008;24(Suppl. 1):S34–S39

24. Taylor LM Jr, Porter JM. The clinical course of diabetics who require emergent foot surgery because of infection or ischemia. *J Vasc Surg* 1987;6:454–459

25. Mills JL, Beckett WC, Taylor SM. The diabetic foot: consequences of delayed treatment and referral. *South Med J* 1991;84:970–974

Suggested Readings

Beach KW, Brunzell JD, Strandness DE Jr. Prevalence of severe arteriosclerosis obliterans in patients with diabetes mellitus: relation to smoking and form of therapy. *Arteriosclerosis* 1982;2:275–280

Goldenberg S, Alex M, Joshi RA, Blumenthal HT. Nonatheromatous peripheral vascular disease of the lower extremity in diabetes mellitus. *Diabetes* 1959;8:261–273

Weitz JI, Byrne J, Clagett GP, et al. Diagnosis and treatment of chronic arterial insufficiency of the lower extremities: a critical review. *Circulation* 1996;94:3026–3049 [erratum 2000;102:1074]

12
Interdisciplinary Team Approach to Targeted Diabetic Foot Care

David G. Armstrong, DPM, MD, PhD[1]; Nicholas Giovinco, DPM[1]; and Joseph L. Mills, MD[2]
[1]University of Arizona College of Medicine, Tucson, AZ; and
[2]Department of Surgery, Baylor College of Medicine, Houston, TX

Limb loss in people with diabetes is a consequence of multifactorial pathology; therefore, it is appropriate to use an interdisciplinary approach to address the specific and varying etiologies that combine to create lower-extremity ulceration, infection, and subsequent amputation.[1] Studies have demonstrated that the 5-year mortality rate in patients with diabetes after major amputation is significant—greater even than many major forms of cancers.[2] More recently, diabetic foot amputations have been compared with landmine-related amputations. This intriguing comparison emphasizes the silent nature of the "warfare" and the sinister consequences on the life of patients/victims. Diabetes around the globe results in one major limb amputation every 30 seconds—that is, over 2,500 limbs lost per day.[3] Therefore, it is vital that appropriate policies be adopted to reduce this epidemic of limb loss.

Team Approach and a Viable Model

A team approach to limb salvage is vital, since no individual medical or surgical specialty is able to manage all aspects of diabetic lower-extremity disease to appropriately manage these patients. Currently, there exists the potential for significant delay between initial patient presentation and subsequent referral between the appropriate medical and surgical specialties. With increased integration among the various specialties that are involved in the care of the

DOI: 10.2337/9781580405706.12

diabetic foot, there is an increased efficiency in rendering care as well as an overall increase in the quality of care provided. Several studies have demonstrated a significant reduction in major amputation rates after development of an interdisciplinary approach to limb salvage and preservation.[4-8]

Diabetic foot ulcerations are progressive in nature and have risk factors such as neuropathy, poor perfusion, and infection, which lead to poor healing and subsequent amputation.[9] Each risk factor is a target for clinical intervention, with the intent to delay or prevent disease progression to amputation. A well-equipped limb salvage team is integral to disease management and must identify, treat, and manage these targets for intervention. The components of the limb salvage team are largely determined by the major pathology noted at presentation. It is our experience that the irreducible minimum for such an interdisciplinary approach be founded in a team that is composed at its core of, first, clinicians caring for the structural and surgical aspects of the foot (podiatric surgeons) and, second, clinicians caring for the vascular interventions into the foot (vascular surgeons). However, the comprehensive care model includes expertise from primary care, diabetology, infectious disease, physical therapy, plastic surgery, nursing, emergency medicine, and prosthetics. Figure 12.1 illustrates a typical limb-salvage team structure and the interdisciplinary components.

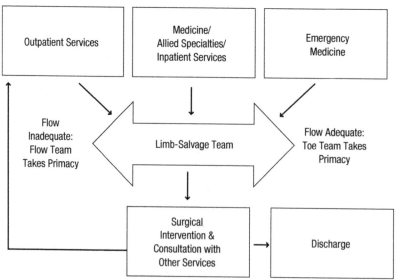

Figure 12.1—Limb salvage team structure and interdisciplinary management.

Both vasculopathy and neuropathy are critical contributors to diabetic foot ulceration.[10] Therefore, it is appropriate to use an interdisciplinary team approach to address specifically the varying factors that combine to create lower-extremity ulceration, infection, and subsequent amputation. Such interdisciplinary models were demonstrated to be highly effective in reducing the incidence of nontraumatic amputations in the diabetic population. A search of the literature reveals that little has been published on the requisite skillsets of the interdisciplinary team to promote limb preservation in patients with diabetes. To that end, a recent article addressing the essential components introduced the diabetic rapid response acute foot team (DRRAFT).[1] This example is an interdisciplinary team model in which the core involves the ability to diagnose rapidly and provide effective treatment to patients with lower-extremity complications of diabetes, using seven basic skillsets. The "irreducible minimum" regarding interdisciplinary units must be oriented around treatment teams that are staffed by members of the podiatric surgery (toe component) and vascular surgery (flow component) specialties, with adjunctive team members being added as necessary via judicious use of consultation. The DRRAFT concept is the natural extension of this premise: bringing the nuances from each individual specialty, the team collectively must possess the ability to perform seven essential skills to be effective in promoting limb preservation. However, any clinician involved in the care of the diabetic patient with a passion for limb salvage can function as a member of the DRRAFT limb-salvage team. Indeed, often, geographic limitation will require that requisite team member roles be performed by physicians trained in global wound care, advanced practice nurses, or clinical nurse specialists. The seven components for the DRRAFT model are presented in Table 12.1. These skillsets were further refined into an American Diabetes Association (ADA) consensus document focusing on inpatient management of diabetic foot complications.[11]

The Interdisciplinary Pathway

In the interdisciplinary limb-salvage model proposed, patients present to a clinic that ideally is staffed by both podiatric and vascular surgeons. On presentation, patients are evaluated using the ADA comprehensive foot examination and risk assessment criteria.[12] Patients are screened and stratified according to risk based on history, dermatologic examination, evaluation of neuropathy, vascular assessment, and biomechanical assessment (Table 12.2). Those patients

Table 12.1 Seven Essential Skills for Effective Limb Preservation: The DRRAFT Team

1. The ability to perform hemodynamic and anatomic vascular assessment with revascularization, as necessary.
2. The ability to perform neurologic workup.
3. The ability to perform site-appropriate culture technique.
4. The ability to perform wound assessment and staging/grading of infection and ischemia.
5. The ability to perform site-specific bedside and intraoperative incision and debridement.
6. The ability to initiate and modify culture-specific and patient-appropriate antibiotic therapy.
7. The ability to perform appropriate postoperative monitoring to reduce risks of reulceration and infection.

who are found to be at increased risk (i.e., patients with current ulcerations or with a history of ulceration, patients with impaired vascular status, or patients who present with lower-extremity deformity) are noted and immediately receive further workup, with an emphasis on timely intervention.[12–15] In the model proposed, those patients who present with diabetic foot ulcers are classified according to the wound, ischemia, and foot infection (WIFI) classification (see Chapter 11) and are immediately sent for a thorough vascular workup including noninvasive vascular studies.[16,17] Invasive vascular intervention, such as endovascular procedures or open bypass, follows as necessary to increase lower-extremity tissue perfusion. In this model, podiatric surgical intervention may take the form of debridement before revascularization attempts, as in the case of significant soft tissue infection, osteomyelitis, or abscess, as well surgical reconstructive efforts after the requisite revascularization and subsequent preventive offloading after limb-salvage attempts. In addition to surgical intervention in the acute setting, podiatric surgery provides continuing lower-extremity wound care to those patients who present with nonischemic wounds, or to those patients whose existing comorbidities limit surgical intervention. After all salvage efforts, the patients are followed according to the current ADA risk classification follow-up guidelines. Follow-up times diminish as overall risk increases, such that those patients in risk category 3 (individuals with previous history of ulceration or amputation) are seen at frequent intervals—no less than every 1–2 months.

After initial intervention and subsequent limb preservation, a strong policy of prevention of reulceration is vital to provide continued limb preservation in this high-risk patient population.[12,18,19] As in the acute setting, each element in the proposed interdisciplinary model has roles and responsibilities during the follow-up phase of limb salvage. The vascular surgery component of the team provides continued vascular "surveillance" in the postoperative setting to ensure that there is continued patent flow and perfusion into the affected lower extremity, while the podiatric surgery component

Table 12.2 Screening, Classification, and Triage of Diabetic Foot Patients

Priority	Indications	Timeline	Suggested follow-up by specialist
Urgent (active pathology)	Open wound or ulcerative area, with or without signs of infection New neuropathic pain or pain at rest Signs of active Charcot neuroarthropathy (red, hot, swollen midfoot or ankle) Vascular compromise (sudden absence of DP/PT pulses or gangrene)	Immediate referral/consult	As determined by specialist
High (ADA risk category 3)	Presence of diabetes with a previous history of ulcer or lower-extremity amputation	Immediate or "next available" outpatient referral	Every 1–2 months
Moderate (ADA risk category 2)	Peripheral artery disease +/– LOPS DP/PT pulses diminished or absent Presence of swelling or edema	Referral within 1–3 weeks (if not already receiving regular care)	Every 2–3 months
Low (ADA risk category 1)	LOPS +/–longstanding, nonchanging deformity Patient seeks education regarding: foot care, athletic training, appropriate footwear, preventing injury, etc.	Referral within 1–3 months	Annually at minimum

ADA, American Diabetes Association; DP, dorsalis pedis; LOPS, loss of protective sensation; PT, posterior tibial. All patients with diabetes should be seen at least once a year by a foot specialist. Reprinted with permission from Frontline Medical Communications (Miller et al.[20]).

concurrently assists with advanced wound-healing techniques, as necessary, and in the formulation of offloading devices to reduce pressure forces that can stimulate reulceration. It is essential that patients who have some degree of residual foot deformity be fitted for custom-molded devices to appropriately reduce plantar pressures. In addition to the surgical and biomechanical management after limb salvage, it is necessary that the patient maintain strict glycemic control and nutritional status. Rampant hyperglycemia and poor nutritional status will prevent wound healing and will place the patient at increased risk for wound development and regression; therefore, these parameters should be addressed and monitored by the patient's primary care physician or by members of the limb-salvage team.

Toe and Flow

Apart from the improved clinical outcomes associated with an interdisciplinary team approach, there are significant academic and clinical training opportunities that such teams present. In the University of Arizona's Southern Arizona Limb Salvage Alliance (SALSA) model, increased interdisciplinary interaction facilitates communication and enhances perspective among team members, which, in addition to generating improved patient outcomes, allows for significant cross-pollination of clinical knowledge and technique, allowing members of the team to strengthen their clinical decision-making skills and to broaden their medical and surgical skillset. Additionally, it appears that combining these services may help to evolve medical and surgical approaches from reactive and ablative to prophylactic and reconstructive.[22,23] Furthermore, the research opportunities that such interdisciplinary teams present allow for significant advances in the comprehensive management of the diabetic foot and limb preservation, which benefits the health care community overall.

The interdisciplinary approach described by the podiatric surgery/vascular surgery model allows for rapid diagnosis and early access to a variety of treatment options, which generates improved clinical outcomes and leads to an overall decrease in major amputation rates.[1,4] While it is certainly most efficient to have a team that is physically combined, either in the hospital setting or in a tertiary care center, this is not an absolute requirement. A "team" may consist of several physicians and surgeons in a specific geographic area who possess a passion for limb preservation and who use that passion to facilitate rapid referral and transfer of care between specialties as necessary to allow for rapid transition between revascularization efforts and the podiatric surgical intervention that may be required both before and after revascularization.

The interdisciplinary approach with podiatric and vascular surgery as a central "toe and flow" axis to limb salvage appears to be an efficient means for interdisciplinary care and amputation prevention. Patients benefit from simultaneous assessments from podiatric and vascular physicians during the same clinic appointment. This result expedites potential vascular intervention and prevents any unnecessary loss of time in referrals and office visits. Such integrative teams allow for increased communication and perspective among team members, which fosters a spirit of learning and exchange of ideas that benefits both patients and team members.

References

1. Fitzgerald RH, Mills JL, Joseph W, Armstrong DG. The diabetic rapid response acute foot team: 7 essential skills for targeted limb salvage. *Eplasty* 2009;9:e15

2. Armstrong DG, Wrobel J, Robbins JM. Guest editorial: are diabetes-related wounds and amputations worse than cancer? *Int Wound J* 2007; 4:286–287

3. Bharara M, Mills JL, Suresh K, et al. Diabetes and landmine-related amputations: a call to arms to save limbs. *Int Wound J* 2009;6:2–3

4. Van Gils CC, Wheeler LA, Mellstrom M, et al. Amputation prevention by vascular surgery and podiatry collaboration in high-risk diabetic and nondiabetic patients: the Operation Desert Foot experience. *Diabetes Care* 1999;22:678–683

5. Frykberg RG. Team approach toward lower extremity amputation prevention in diabetes. *J Am Podiatr Med Assoc* 1997;87:305–312

6. Canavan RJ, Unwin NC, Kelly WF, Connolly VM. Diabetes- and nondiabetes-related lower extremity amputation incidence before and after the introduction of better organized diabetes foot care: continuous longitudinal monitoring using a standard method. *Diabetes Care* 2008;31:459–463

7. Krishnan S, Nash F, Baker N, et al. Reduction in diabetic amputations over 11 years in a defined U.K. population: benefits of multidisciplinary team work and continuous prospective audit. *Diabetes Care* 2008; 31:99–101

8. Larsson J, Eneroth M, Apelqvist J, Stenstrom A. Sustained reduction in major amputations in diabetic patients: 628 amputations in 461 patients in a defined population over a 20-year period. *Acta Orthop* 2008; 79:665–673

9. Larsson J, Apelqvist J, Agardh CD, Stenstrom A. Decreasing incidence of major amputation in diabetic patients: a consequence of a multidisciplinary foot care team approach? *Diabet Med* 1995;12:770–776

10. Pecoraro RE, Reiber GE, Burgess EM. Pathways to diabetic limb amputation: basis for prevention. *Diabetes Care* 1990;13:513–521

11. Wukich DK, Armstrong DG, Attinger CE, et al. Inpatient management of diabetic foot disorders: a clinical guide. *Diabetes Care* 2013;36; 2862–2871

12. Boulton AJ, Armstrong DG, Albert SF, et al. Comprehensive foot examination and risk assessment: a report of the task force of the foot care interest group of the American Diabetes Association, with endorsement by the American Association of Clinical Endocrinologists. *Diabetes Care* 2008;31:1679–1685

13. Armstrong DG, Lavery LA, Harkless LB. Validation of a diabetic wound classification system: the contribution of depth, infection, and ischemia to risk of amputation. *Diabetes Care* 1998;21:855–859

14. Lavery LA, Armstrong DG, Vela SA, et al. Practical criteria for screening patients at high risk for diabetic foot ulceration. *Arch Intern Med* 1998;158:158–162

15. Lavery LA, Armstrong DG, Wunderlich RP, et al. Risk factors for foot infections in individuals with diabetes. *Diabetes Care* 2006;29:1288–1293

16. Mills JL Sr, Conte MS, Armstrong DG, et al. The Society of Vasulcar Surgery Lower Extremity Threatened Limb Classification System: Risk stratification based on wound, ischemia and foot infection (WIfI). *J Vasc Surg* 2014;59:220–234

17. Cull DL, Manos G, Hartley MC, et al. An early validation of the Society for Vascular Surgery lower extremity threatened limb classification system. *J Vasc Surg* 2014;60:1535–1541

18. Wu SC, Crews RT, Armstrong DG. The pivotal role of offloading in the management of neuropathic foot ulceration. *Curr Diab Rep* 2005; 5:423–429

19. Lavery LA, Wunderlich RP, Tredwell JL. Disease management for the diabetic foot: effectiveness of a diabetic foot prevention program to reduce amputations and hospitalizations. *Diabetes Res Clin Pract* 2005; 70:31–37

20. Miller JD, Carter E, Shih J, et al. How to do a 3-minute diabetic foot exam. *J Fam Pract* 2014;63:646–656

21. Boulton AJ, Armstrong DG, Albert SF, et al. Comprehensive foot examination and risk assessment: a report of the task force of the foot care interest group of the American Diabetes Association, with endorsement by the American Association of Clinical Endocrinologists. *Diabetes Care* 2008;31:1679–1685

22. Armstrong DG, Bharara M, White M, et al. The impact and outcomes of establishing an integrated interdisciplinary surgical team to care for the diabetic foot. *Diabetes Metab Res Rev* 2012;28:514–518

23. Chung J, Modrall JG, Ahn C, et al. Multidisciplinary care improves amputation-free survival in patients with chronic critical limb ischemia. *J Vasc Surg* 2015;61:162–169 doi:10.1016/j.jvs.2014.05.101. Epub 2014 Sept 8

Index